T0258906

Medical Humanities Com

VOLUME ONE

Medical Humanities Companion
VOLUME ONE

Symptom

Edited by
Martyn Evans
Rolf Ahlzén
Iona Heath
and
Jane Macnaughton

Series Editors
Rolf Ahlzén, Martyn Evans, Pekka Louhiala
and Raimo Puustinen

Radcliffe Publishing
Oxford • New York

Radcliffe Publishing Ltd
18 Marcham Road
Abingdon
Oxon OX14 1AA
United Kingdom

www.radcliffe-oxford.com

Electronic catalogue and worldwide online ordering facility.

British Library Cataloguing in Publication Data

A catalogue record for this book is available from the British Library.

ISBN-13: 978 184619 286 9

Typeset by Pindar NZ, Auckland, New Zealand

Contents

About the series editors

Rolf Ahlzén is working part-time as a general practitioner outside Karlstad in south-west Sweden. He is also the chairman of the ethical committee in the region of Värmland. He holds a position as senior lecturer in public health at Karlstad University, focusing mainly on healthcare ethics and on the history of ideas and science.

Martyn Evans joined Durham University in 2002 as Professor of Humanities in Medicine and Principal of John Snow College, and became Principal of Trevelyan College in 2008. He taught philosophy and ethics of medicine at the University of Wales for several years.

He was founding joint editor of the *Medical Humanities* edition of the *Journal of Medical Ethics* from 2000 to 2008. He has published variously on the aesthetics of music, ethics and philosophy of medicine, and the role of humanities in medical education. His current interests include music and medicine, the nature and role of humanities in medicine, and philosophical problems in medicine. In 2005 he was made an honorary Fellow of the Royal College of General Practitioners.

Pekka Louhiala is a lecturer in medical ethics at the University of Helsinki, Finland. He has degrees in both medicine and philosophy, and he also works as a part-time paediatrician in private practice. He has published on various topics in medical ethics, philosophy of medicine and epidemiology. His current academic interests include conceptual and philosophical issues in medicine, such as evidence-based medicine and placebo effects.

Raimo Puustinen is a full-time general practitioner and a senior consultant at Pihlajalinna Medical Centre, Tampere, Finland. He has published articles and books on general practice, medical ethics and philosophy of medicine. When not practising medicine or contemplating theoretical issues in medical practice, he plays jazz on the tenor saxophone. He is married, and has four children and two grandchildren.

List of contributors

Jill Gordon
Honorary Associate Professor, Centre for Values Ethics and the Law in Medicine, University of Sydney

Iona Heath
General practitioner, Kentish Town, London

Anne MacLeod
Dermatologist and writer from the North of Scotland

Jane Macnaughton
Director of the Centre for Arts and Humanities in Health and Medicine (CAHHM)
Clinical Senior Lecturer, Durham University

Carl-Edvard Rudebeck
Research Adviser, Kalmar County Council
Professor, Institute for Community Medicine, Tromsö University, Norway
General practitioner, Esplanaden Health Centre, Västervik

John Saunders
Honorary Professor, Centre for Philosophy, Humanities and Law in Healthcare, School of Health Science, University of Wales, Swansea
Honorary Senior Lecturer, College of Medicine, University of Wales, Cardiff
Consultant Physician, Nevill Hall Hospital, Abergavenny

Acknowledgements

The Editors wish to thank the Nuffield Trust and the University of Wales for making possible, at the magnificent Gregynog Hall in Powys, Wales, the academic seminar that first led us on to the path of collaborative publication. We are enormously grateful to Gillian Nineham, Managing Editor of Radcliffe Publishing, for personally encouraging the publication of an initial volume of philosophical writings on clinical practice, and then for seeing through the 'lens' of that volume the possibilities of a fuller medical humanities series. The subsequent support of Radcliffe Publishing was crucial for the development of the series, particularly at our first interdisciplinary planning meeting at Radcliffe's Abingdon headquarters.

We are indebted to all of our fellow contributors who between them also provided a considerable amount of mutual peer review. Special mention must be made of one of these contributors, Raimo Puustinen, whose many talents included finding the Villa Belpoggio in Tuscany, the ideal location for the book conference which led to this volume. Raimo alone had the foresight to bring his family with him to that idyllic spot. The rest of us therefore owe correspondingly even greater debts of gratitude to our own families, who have supported our participation in the project despite forgoing the pleasures of a truly inspirational location.

Finally, we would like to record particular thanks to Maria Ventrone, who oversaw our hospitality in the Villa Belpoggio with thoughtful insight into the nature of the project that we were attempting, and whose abundant humanity had helped her to overcome her own serious illness in a way that gave us real inspiration. This volume is respectfully and affectionately dedicated to her.

Introduction

Falling ill is not something that happens to us, it is a choice we make as
a result of things happening to us. It is an action we take when we feel
unacceptably odd. Obviously, there are times when this choice is taken
out of the victim's hands: he may be so overwhelmed by events that he
plays no active part in what happens next and is brought to the doctor
by friends or relatives, stricken and helpless. But this is rare. Most people
who fall ill have chosen to cast themselves in the role of patient. Viewing
their unfortunate situation, they see themselves as sick people and begin
to act differently.

Jonathan Miller[1]

'. . . when we feel unacceptably odd' – this is a curious yet perceptive description
of the onset of a symptom, the point at which we notice in our self-experience
something that is both different and unwelcome, both odd and, in the long
run, unacceptable. It is with such unacceptable oddness, such unwanted
intrusions into our self-awareness marking the first stages of illness, that this
book is concerned. In it we shall attempt to explore the idea of symptoms,
their experiential reality, and their significance. However, this is not a clinical
textbook, nor is it an anthropological survey, or a historical review. If it were
any single thing, one might perhaps say that it was a somewhat fictionalised
form of doing philosophy. But what this means is really the attempt to bring
both reason and imagination to bear on the question of how symptoms are
to be understood.

In attempting this, we are really only making explicit something – the
imagination – that is intimately involved in most forms of reasoning anyway,
however un-obvious that might sometimes be. As Jonathan Miller (with whose
shrewd observation we began) himself put it, in the development of medico-

scientific understanding of the human body, 'the most impressive contribution to the growth of intelligibility has been made by the application of suggestive metaphors.'[2] The heart as a pump is comprehensible enough. Voluntary muscular movement as the operation of automatic gun turrets is perhaps less so. However, between these the physiological counterparts of 'furnaces, crucibles, ovens, hearths, retorts and stills' and devices which 'lift, dig, hoist, wind, pump, press, filter and extract'[3] provide a wealth of analogies that have enabled medicine 'to visualise the body not merely as an intelligible system, but as an organised system of systems – which does not mean that man is an engine or that his humanity is a delusion.'[4] Miller's concern is to counter the popular rejection of science, or at least that form of rejection which supposes science to be destructive of the human imagination, and in this he is surely right. However, his method is a challenging one – namely to show 'that one of the most effective ways of restoring and preserving man's humanity is by acknowledging the extent to which he is a material mechanism.'[5]

This is of course itself a further, very large metaphor. Indeed, it is an important part of medical science's contemporary organising metaphor for human nature. This is a metaphor to be taken seriously, not least by those who find it ultimately unsatisfying. And the notion of a symptom is as good a starting point as any, for trying to take seriously the extraordinary fusion of the material and the existential that is conscious human experience. Nowhere is this more important than in health and sickness, and in our organised responses to the challenges of both.

WHAT WE ARE TRYING TO DO: WHAT WE TAKE MEDICAL HUMANITIES TO BE, AND TO ATTEMPT

The phrase 'medical humanities' has a currency that is perhaps wider than any agreement as to what it means. Even so, those engaged in medical humanities usually know what they are attempting. In Volume One we are attempting to understand the very *idea* of a symptom, and also the implications of particular symptoms. The idea of a symptom is important for understanding the structure of clinical practice. However, the particularity of specific symptoms is important for understanding the fact that real, actual symptoms are always experienced by real, actual individuals – however much those experiences are mediated by language, culture, expectation and the conventions of the clinical consultation. And this in turn is important because it reminds us that health, illness, well-being and suffering are first and foremost aspects of experience.

Scientific medicine describes the material substances of health and illness, but the reason why patients consult their doctors is generally because something is amiss in their experiences of daily living. Inflammation is significant to patients not in itself but because of the felt soreness, stiffness or visible disfigurement that it produces. Low blood pressure may be privately applauded by doctors even though their patients complain of feeling dizzy if they get up too quickly. A blocked Fallopian tube is of only theoretical interest to the patient, until she feels the despair of being unable to conceive a longed-for child. Medical humanities perspectives on symptoms and 'the symptom' pay special attention to these experiential aspects because, in the end, it is these experiential aspects that motivate people to go and seek help from medicine and healthcare.

TAKING SUBJECTIVITY SERIOUSLY

How are such experiential aspects to be understood, reckoned with and incorporated into clinical understanding? It is necessary somehow to take seriously the patient's *subjectivity*. This means taking seriously the content of the patient's individual point of view, the way of life that has led up to it, the meanings and connotations that inform it, and the way it is shaped by other people – including, of course, the clinician. From the perspective of clinical understanding and decision making, this means taking the thoughts and attitudes of the patient-in-context as seriously as the generalised truths about the human organism supplied by the natural sciences. The natural sciences give us knowledge that defines the boundaries of rational conceptions of what people might do. However, we look elsewhere – to the humanities and social sciences – to understand the basis of people's attitudes towards what they *should* do, and their motives for what they in fact do.[6]

THE IDEA OF THE PATIENT'S PROGRESS

In looking at symptoms, and at the idea of a symptom, we are in effect charting the first step along the road whereby someone becomes a patient. As we all know, into every life some rain must fall, and as we equally well know, this rain sometimes takes the form of illness, infirmity or disability. The first drops of rain are the symptoms – the growing awareness that something is not right, that something unwanted and unbidden is happening, something that is unwanted in itself and also unwanted because of what it might lead to.

What happens thereafter depends on many things – the seriousness of the underlying reason for the symptom, the patient's tolerance of non-serious illnesses, the availability of accessible healthcare, and so on – and we shall explore these sequels in future volumes. However, for now our attention is focused on this first phenomenon – the symptom. Depending on what happens, it may successfully be ignored and never amount to anything else. Alternatively, it may turn out to be the forerunner of catastrophe.

Only later, looking backwards – perhaps from the other side of illness, diagnosis, treatment, and maybe recovery – will the symptom take its place as the opening event in a full sequence of events, a story that is played out in the life of a particular human being, the patient. At the outset, we do not even know whether the symptom will form a part of any subsequent story at all.

We do know, however, what might count as a story. In his extraordinary autobiographical account of a severe leg injury, neurologist Oliver Sacks tells at least two stories about his illness, recovery and convalescence.[7] One story – in the sense of a structured sequence of events in time, linked in terms that are at least partly causal – concerns the 'career' of the pathology within his leg in terms of the fragmentation and reconstruction of human tissue even at the cellular level. It has its narrative sequence, its cast of characters and – for the onlooker – its high stakes and its dramatic suspense. But of course this is in real terms only a parallel set of phenomena to the story that matters – the 'career' of the sufferer, the immobilised and frustrated mountain climber, the fearful yet curious medically qualified patient. And we can say that this is the story that matters because the cellular 'story' takes its interest from the *existential implications* it has for Sacks, the sufferer, the man, whereas the patient's story consists precisely in those existential implications.

DISCIPLINES, ENQUIRIES AND QUESTIONS

This book might have been very different had we pursued our original intention of producing a series of volumes each tied to a separate disciplinary viewpoint. A number of the contributors had previously collaborated on just such a volume, self-consciously collecting together, and bringing to bear upon clinical medicine, aspects of enquiry within a single humanities discipline, namely philosophy.[8] It might have been possible therefore to repeat that exercise for other humanities disciplines, such as medical history, literature studies, linguistics or art theory, or for social sciences disciplines, such as anthropology or sociology. However, the ready availability of this approach perhaps suggested that it was not sufficiently fresh.

An alternative method, that of bringing together different disciplinary viewpoints *simultaneously* to bear on a common object of enquiry – insofar as this can be done – seemed both more ambitious and more attractive.[9] More attractive, because a series of volumes each looking at a different stage in the sequence of stages of the illness process would accumulate into a larger overall story, a story that could be followed in both narrative and analytic form, and because many different kinds of voices would be heard within each volume. Each volume would be a kaleidoscope in itself.

But more ambitious, too – because the very idea of a 'common object of enquiry' becomes fragile when we look at something through very different disciplinary perspectives. If the disciplines are sufficiently far apart – consider, say, religious studies and genetics – then it is obvious enough that the theologian on the one hand and the molecular biologist on the other do not really see the same thing when they look at the vulnerable human being. However, even more closely related disciplines *within* the aegis of the humanities may vary as well in terms of their perspective. Is an illness *as an object of enquiry* necessarily the same thing for the philosopher as for the historian? At any rate, the question certainly arises, and we are under no illusions about the task ahead if we are to make Volume One and its later companions a genuine fusion of disciplinary insights, discourses and metaphors.[10]

In Volume One, our hope is to ask questions about the meaning of actual symptoms and of the concept 'symptom', from a convergent range of disciplinary expertise, as the prelude to a cumulative interdisciplinary understanding of illness as a human need, and clinical medicine as a human response to it.

THE STORIES

We have structured our thoughts around the symptoms encountered by four representative, albeit fictionalised, patients. Their varied stories derive from actual clinical experiences, but are sufficiently removed from identifiable individuals as to avoid questions of consent or anonymity. Between them, Rachel, Jake, Liz and Jen represent a variety of ages, symptom experiences and types of underlying clinical condition, although we recognise that they fall within a common cultural milieu. They are imagined and described for us by a published novelist and poet who is also a specialist physician working in dermatology, and who combines reason and imagination in both of her chosen professions.

The onset of symptoms is of course only the first stage in the journey undertaken by a patient. In subsequent volumes we shall follow these four patients on the successive stages of their journeys.

THE WRITERS

A few years ago a number of us met in an old country house in rural Wales to consider how we might pursue the virtues of philosophical and other forms of humanities study in an understanding of medicine and healthcare. It might be said that what prompted our original conversations were our various species of dissatisfaction with the ways in which clinical medicine was being analysed, researched, taught and – in some ways – practised. From the outset, several different disciplines and a number of nations were represented. Today we comprise medical specialists, general medical practitioners and humanities scholars from Australia, England, Finland, Scotland, Sweden and Wales. We share a determination to pursue our fictional patients along their respective journeys, which – as we look ahead – will lead them to their different clinical consultations, history takings, diagnoses, treatments and, for better or worse, eventual outcomes. We do not know exactly where our patients' journeys will lead them, nor where our own enquiries will lead *us*. However, we hope to accompany them to their destinations, and we hope that our readers in turn will accompany us.

Martyn Evans, Rolf Ahlzén, Iona Heath and Jane Macnaughton
September 2008

REFERENCES

1 Miller J. *The Body in Question*. London: Jonathan Cape Ltd; 1978. p. 49.
2 Ibid., p. 9.
3 Ibid., p. 10.
4 Ibid., p. 10.
5 Ibid., pp. 10–11.
6 Evans HM. Medical humanities: stranger at the gate, or long-lost friend? *Med Health Care Philos*. 2007; **10**: 363–72.
7 Sacks O. *A Leg to Stand On*. New York: Touchstone; 1998.
8 Evans M, Louhiala P, Puustinen R. *Philosophy for Medicine: applications in a clinical context*. Oxford: Radcliffe Publishing; 2004.
9 We are grateful to Dr Neil Pickering, University of Otago, who thoughtfully drew our attention to this fundamental alternative early on in this project.
10 Evans HM, Macnaughton RJ. Should medical humanities be a multidisciplinary or an interdisciplinary study? *J Med Ethics: Med Humanities*. **30**: 1–4.

The patients' stories: Rachel, Jake, Liz and Jen

ANNE MACLEOD

RACHEL, 10 YEARS OLD

It started one Thursday last autumn. I know it was a Thursday, I didn't want to go to orchestra. Mum never lets me miss it.

'Put your violin in the car, Rachel.' She was busy unpacking the weekly shop. She'd been to the newest, cheapest supermarket. Bought oceans of apple juice. The cupboard would be swimming in it.

'Can we take one of those cartons? I'm thirsty.' I grabbed one.

'Leave them alone! And get that violin in the boot. Did you practise at all this week? I didn't hear you.'

'I hate orchestra.'

'No, you don't!' Mum looked at me, carefully, as if she hadn't seen me in a long time. 'You seem a bit peaky. What's up?'

'What's up?' I shouted. 'I'm too tired to go out. I want to go to bed!'

'You want to go to bed?' She could not believe her ears.

'I'm exhausted. Fed up. Starving!' I was crying now.

'You can't be starving. You just scoffed half a packet of Jaffa Cakes!'

I stomped over to the sink and ran the cold tap. Filled a glass. Filled it too high.

'Rachel! Watch what you're doing.'

I slurped till it was safe to lift the glass, then drank the water quickly, all in one, which left me even more thirsty. That was the funny thing – I couldn't remember the last time I didn't feel thirsty.

'Go and get –' Mum was interrupted by the front door creaking. 'Rachel! We're so late. That's Leroy home already!'

I raced from the room. Not to fetch the violin, but to slip into the loo before my brother could get in and start his endless showering. He was going on a date, and it always takes him hours to get ready. I just got there before him. He thumped the door.

'Get out of there! Rachel! Mum – tell her I need in!'

I could hear Mum sighing. She went on unpeeling the shopping from the mountain of carrier bags.

'Leroy!' she shouted. 'Where did you put the stuff I bought last week for the party? Blackberry water, apple water. There should be four bottles.'

Leroy sounded puzzled. 'I put them in the larder, like you said.'

'You didn't.'

'Course I did. Where else would I put them? They don't fit in the cupboards. I bet Rachel's swiped the lot.' He stomped upstairs, making for my room.

I sat in the bathroom, shivering. Feeling sick. I'd been feeling sick all day. He'd find them. I knew Mum would be mad, but I couldn't help it. I'd been so thirsty. Didn't mean to drink them all.

Not that the water helped. I'd been up all night, running to the loo. Every night. I'd been running to the loo for days and days. Weeks and weeks. Always, always thirsty.

'Mum!' Leroy was stomping down the stairs now, two empty plastic bottles under each arm. I couldn't carry them like that and nor could my brother. He dropped them. The bottles rattled down the stairs. Good thing they were plastic. 'Look, Mum,' he seemed surprised. As if he couldn't understand. 'They're empty – all empty. Every single one.'

Next thing, he and Mum were both rapping the door, shoving it, but I had the lock on. I felt sick and cold, and far too tired to move. I'd been tired for so long.

I was shivering, sweating. Wouldn't move. Couldn't. No way. I'd only need the loo again. They'd just have to wait.

For a long time they went on knocking and shouting, sounding further and further away. I was sick, actually sick. I've never felt so dizzy.

I lay down on the floor. Maybe I fell.

That's when the room went dark.

JAKE, 27 YEARS OLD

'You coming to the pool?'

'Maybe next week,' Jake tried to smile at Carol, not that that was hard. He would have smiled at her day and night, given half a chance. It wasn't often that their shifts coincided.

'Izzy tells me you were the best swimmer in your school. Won medals. Swam for Scotland.'

'Izzy talks too much.'

Carol shook her head. 'Sure you won't come?'

'Sorry, something on.' Jake watched her walk away, linking arms with Izzy and Jon.

'What d'you think you're doing?' Frank was standing behind him.

'What d'you mean?'

'I've seen how you look at that girl. Why chase her away? She was chatting you up. That's the nearest she'll get to asking you out, and you blew it.'

Jake blushed.

'No sense in playing hard to get,' Frank rumbled on. 'She'll think you're not interested. When I was your age . . .' the lecture went on and on. Jake quite liked Frank, but sometimes the old night porter talked too much. 'You mustn't do yourself down,' Frank finished. 'It's not the end of the world, after all.'

'What isn't?' Jake hadn't been paying attention.

'The skin. The psoriasis.'

Jake couldn't believe his ears. He blushed redder than the roses on the high reception desk.

'Like they say,' Frank shook his head, 'there's a lot of it about.'

The walk back to his flat should have taken no longer than ten minutes. Fifteen at most. Tonight, Jake took the scenic route, lingering by the river, staring down into the squirming darkness of the waves. He stood so long that the homeless guys below the bridge clanked their bottles, laughing.

'Make up your mind!' they taunted. 'Go on. Jump!'

Jake ignored them, like he tried to ignore the couple kissing across the street. If that were him and Carol –

'Can't you do it for yourself?' the male half of the couple was moving towards him, aggressive.

'Sorry, mate,' Jake backed away. 'Didn't mean to stare.'

Had he been staring? He sprinted for home, the second-storey flat he had been so proud to find. It wasn't exactly posh, but it was central, and it was his. Somehow he managed the mortgage payments. A place of his own. Privacy. His own door. His own shower.

It was dark in the stairwell, the light bulb blown. Why did that happen so often? He'd have to change it tomorrow before old Mrs Anderson had a go. He didn't want her falling again.

Maybe he should change it tonight? It was pitch black, so black you couldn't see your hand in front of your face. You couldn't see where to put your feet.

He found himself falling suddenly, tripping over something soft huddled on his doorstep. The something yelped.

'Jake?'

'Carol? What the – what are you doing here?'

'Being a doormat,' she sighed. 'Aren't you going to ask me in?'

They picked themselves up slowly. Jake was silent, tongue-tied.

Carol took charge. 'Well, now,' she said, 'Coffee? Glass of wine? You were going to ask me in, right?'

Jake cleared his throat, nodded. 'I'll put the kettle on.' Was the flat tidy? Was the kitchen clean? 'Come in.' Even as he spoke, even as he filled the kettle, he could feel the early crampings in his gut.

No! Not again. Not now. Any minute he'd be bent double. 'Carol,' he mumbled through the lancing pain. 'Can you take over here?'

He reached the bathroom just in time. Emerging, shamefaced, he found her sitting on the sofa. She'd switched on the CD player. She'd dimmed the lights.

'If I didn't know better,' she said, 'I'd think I wasn't welcome.'

Jake didn't know what to say. The gut let him down more and more often. Greasy food, the slightest stress –

She broke the silence.

'I know better. Come here, you daft thing. *Now.*'

LIZ, 30-SOMETHING

It was raining out, raining heavily. Liz had, of course, forgotten her umbrella. And she hadn't worn her raincoat. The plan had been to come home before the clinic, take a shower, do a little light shopping en route. Retail therapy. She hated the annual ceremony of the smear – which was how she thought of it, in an effort to diminish the intrusion. Not that the nurses weren't nice, and perfectly professional. They did what they could to limit the indignity, the humiliation of it all. Liz couldn't help feeling humiliated. It was how she felt. Invaded. It always seemed such an alien encounter. Those high, narrow couches. The rasping paper. The hardness of the thing they poked inside you. And then the interminable wait for the result.

That was how it went in a good year. Indignity regraded. Reassured. Everything to plan. Today, though, nothing had gone to plan. She should have stayed in bed this morning, turned over, gone back to sleep, cancelled her appointment. Taken a duvet day. She'd had the headache from the start.

Not the aura though.

She flopped on the sofa, light-headed.

'Mum, are you all right?'

'I'm fine, Sophie. Fine.'

'You don't look fine.'

She shook her head. 'It's only the rain. What are you watching?'

'*Neighbours.*'

'Soph! I wish you wouldn't.'

'You always say that, Mum!'

'It's for the brain-dead.'

'You only think that because you're older than the hills.'

'Thank you very much!' Liz stared into the distance. She still felt cold. A shower perhaps? Yes, a shower might help. She pulled herself to her feet. She hadn't felt like this for weeks. Months, maybe. If she could just get warm . . . She made it to the bedroom. Lowered herself on to the bed. *When you're feeling that way*, she could hear her mother hectoring, *sit down or lie down. Lying is better. If you can.*

Oh I can, the young Liz laughed to herself. *Lying. Yes, I certainly can. Like a trooper.* The lies she had told! To get out, to be free, to be independent, somehow, of her parents. To forget the label.

Epileptic.

But lying down, now, seemed like a good idea. Had she taken her medication? It had been so long since she had one turn, never mind two. Coming round on the practice couch, to the nurse's shocked and somehow apologetic stare, she had found herself in post-fit confusion. Her memory, her sense of direction, even her speech, wouldn't be right for days. Had she taken her medication this morning? Had she? She couldn't remember.

The worry of the smear, and then Carlos phoning, disrupted her determinedly calm routine. Was that what had set this off? The worry of the smear? Or Carlos muscling in? Had he been muscling in? Was she confusing now with then, those early days of separation, days when Carlos and his lawyer insinuated – insisted – that she could not cope with a small child?

Lie flat, her mother droned, *on your side. Have someone with you.*

There'd been no one for so long. No one but Sophie. Perhaps, Liz wondered, drifting, perhaps this would pass.

It sometimes did.

JEN, 70 YEARS OLD

'That'll be the post, Jen. The post!'

'Just going, Geoff.' Jen struggled to keep her voice bright. It wasn't Geoff's fault that he couldn't get to the door. The impatience, the obsessions, the overwhelming need to have things done by yesterday – none of these were his fault either, hard though they might be to live with. Before the stroke, Geoff had been a different man. Jen told herself this every day – ten times every day. It didn't really make life easier.

The doorbell rang again.

'Jen! That'll be the post!'

This time she didn't answer, but opened the door.

'Morning, Harry.'

'Is it Harry?' Geoff's voice nagged in the background. 'Is it Harry, Jen?'

'Lively today,' said Harry, handing over a pile of envelopes. 'You're looking a bit peaky, though. Got to look after yourself, Mrs D. Don't want to be catching that bird-flu they're all on about.'

'No. Thanks,' Jen smiled. 'You take care, Harry.'

She was tired today. No energy. Moving through the rooms she had polished and tended so carefully for 40 years – 40 years! – Jen's hands shook.

'Was it Harry? Jen! Was it Harry? Is it the post, Jen? Bring it here.'

'I'm coming, Geoff.' She couldn't shout. Couldn't manage more than a whisper.

'What's come today? What have we got?'

Jen had already sorted through the mail. Bills, advertisements, a letter from Jane. And a brown envelope addressed in a childish hand to Mrs J Doughty. The postmark told her it had been franked at the Royal Infirmary. Jen felt her knees grow weaker. She felt dizzy. Her heart raced. Dr Gaitens had said the appointment would come within the week, but she had translated that to weeks, perhaps months.

'We can't ignore it. Coughing blood is something we have to investigate,' he'd smiled, and Jen tried to feel looked after. 'You've lost a bit of weight. Have you been dieting?'

'Not hungry, doctor,' Jen sighed.

In the next room, Geoff called out, 'Jen! Is that Dr Gaitens? Is he coming in?'

'Are you coping?' Dr Gaitens knew exactly how hard it was to get through a day with Geoff.

Jen smiled, didn't answer.

The antibiotics he had given her didn't seem to do much but give her diarrhoea. Every morning, the first cough brought a smear of blood. She burned the tissues. What if it was TB? What then?

'You'll have to tell him,' Dr Gaitens had been firm. 'You'll have to tell him you've an appointment at the hospital. That you're not feeling so good. We'll organise some help.'

'He wouldn't have it,' said Jen. 'I'll try the tablets. See how it goes.'

Dr Gaitens shook his head. 'You'll have your appointment within the week. When did you stop smoking?'

And here it was. How could a slip of paper seem so heavy?

'Jen! Where are you? Where's my post?'

Post. Right. Jen pulled herself up to her full height. Straightened her shoulders.

'Coming, Geoff.' She tucked the envelope in her pocket.

CHAPTER 1

Music, interrupted: an illness observed from within

MARTYN EVANS

COLDNESS

It is 4.20 on a soot-black November morning. Outside, in a few hours dawn will reveal a hard frost crystallising the ground and turning grass leaves into spears. The air temperature is 4 or 5 degrees below zero. Indoors, the room has settled at what ought to be a more comfortable 8 degrees for sleeping, but despite the coolness sleep eludes me anyway.

For who can sleep in the grip of these dreadful hot-cold flushes/sweats/shivers? For some reason I can attain no comfortable constant temperature; the diabolical inner heating dial that lies beneath the implacable grip of my present illness has two exquisitely unstable settings: 'sweat'; 'shiver'. This ought to be no more than the minor misery that it appears when put into words, but from the fragility of my inability to tolerate it I realise that I am, unmistakeably and unambiguously, ill.

But *how* ill? Well, if illness is a first-person matter, if it is the *experience* of something bodily amiss, then the first-person is the best authority concerning the illness's severity: I am as ill as I feel. We men are often reminded by women that our pain thresholds are lower; perhaps this is true for our bodily distress more generally. If with a 'mere cold' a man feels just as ill as a woman feels with influenza, what entitles women to scorn our reported distress? Of course, there is a virological response to this, positively distinguishing the common cold from influenza, and influenza from other respiratory pathogens. Even so, if men simply do in general have a worse experience of a mild pain than do women, wherein lie the facts of the case? Do they lie in some objective external measure of the severity of the painful stimulus, or in the reported intensity of the experience?

Whatever this germ is, knowing its identity would not really dispose of my main concern at this point – the apprehension of symptoms at the time one is having them, and is distressed by them.

SYMPTOMS AND SIGNS TO THE SELF

There is something incomplete about the conventional medical distinction between sign and symptom. The burden of the distinction is between what is in essence a first-hand experience, usually unpleasant – the symptom – and an observed pointer towards something else, something that is *read*, as a sign is 'read' by the doctor, and that points towards something removed from the doctor's first-hand experience, namely the patient's likely future experiences or circumstances. This distinction is a reasonable and helpful one for some practical purposes, but it over-simplifies both doctor and patient. It neglects the first-hand experiential aspect of the doctor's physical senses in her being aware of the signs (and this is a widespread neglect in the popular conventional view of science as being immaculately objective). However, perhaps more importantly, it neglects the patient's appetite for finding *meaning* in what is happening to him. In the process it neglects the patient's own interpretative habits and instincts.

For there is an ambiguity about symptoms and signs. A symptom is also *a sign to the self*, a sign (in the medical sense) that is read by the self, and not by the doctor – at least not initially. If it is publicly visible (for instance, a rash) or, if it is invisible, but then subsequently reported publicly (for instance, persistent nausea), the symptom can become the doctor's sign straightforwardly. But in what context and against what background is it read as a sign by the patient? Against the background, surely, of the taken-for-granted-ness of our ordinary, healthy, non-pathological bodily states and bodily experience. Here, provided that it is not so overwhelming as to leave us no conscious attention for anything else, a symptom automatically alerts us to the fact that something is wrong. It alerts us to look ahead, to the immediate and perhaps also the longer-term future, and to ask ourselves what might await us. However, if a symptom's intensity increases, it can lose this forward-looking aspect for us. A merely quantitative increase in severity can cross a threshold of some kind, producing a qualitative change in the symptom's hold over us.

This, too, is part of its ambiguity. At a low intensity a symptom allows us enough room (or respite) to look ahead. It is as much sign as symptom even for the patient; its sign-ness can be apparent or even dominant. At a sufficiently low intensity, the sign-ness may itself be, or correspond to, something so trivial that the idea of its having any 'meaning' just doesn't arise. At the other extreme, its intensity may be such that the body itself takes charge and 'edits out' the symptom by withdrawing the physiological support for consciousness. Just short of this, the symptom may so fill our consciousness that its sign-ness is lost to view, and 'meaning' simply cannot gain a foothold. At such levels of suffering, the symptom-ness is all that the patient can experience; that the symptom should be made to vanish *now* is all that matters.

FOUR CASES, FIVE PATIENTS

Our quartet of patient stories exhibits well this ambiguity of symptom and sign, and between them these stories also point towards something else which I shall try to explore in this chapter, namely the difference between the simple obstructive or distractive effect of symptoms intruding upon our ordinary daily life (what we might call their noisiness), and the tendency of some sufficiently intense and unpleasant symptoms to capture our consciousness completely (what I shall call their discordance or dys-tone).

For 10-year-old Rachel, her symptoms are both noisy and discordant in the senses that I shall explore. They are also signs of something else that, at her tender age, she cannot readily grasp. The constant thirst and running to the toilet point somewhere, although she probably does not know where. The fact that she predicts the consequences of some of the symptoms is interesting – they point (inductively) to further symptoms. She knows what to expect from constantly taking in fluids; she knows that if she moves from the bathroom she will want the toilet again; she seems to expect to be sick once the sweating and shivering starts. This makes them signs of *something*, but not signs in the medical sense. Tiredness, feeling sick and feeling constantly thirsty obstruct her, but are also intrinsically unpleasant, and this is hardly a matter of gradation for her. We may be able externally to divide up her symptoms in the way that I have suggested, but she is unlikely to do so.

As for 27-year-old Jake, our first clue to his symptoms is given to us by an observer. The night porter, Frank, offers a third-person identification of the more obvious of Jake's symptoms. He gives it its disease-name, psoriasis, but it will be the symptoms that he notices – the inflammation, the encrustation, the weeping of Jake's uncovered skin. These also do duty as signs for the clinician, but they are a kind of sign for the porter as well, of course, and they prompt his advice to Jake not to be beaten by the condition, indicating how he suspects the restrictions that it produces for Jake. Later on we learn of another side to

Jake's misery. His diarrhoea is plainly, for him, both intrinsically unpleasant and socially debilitating, humiliating, a kind of announcement of inadequacy, something which produces the perceived social requirement that he withdraw. It is a symptom of his anxiety, but it also produces anxiety, and he knows it.

Thirty-something Liz has what we might call secondary symptoms or even meta-symptoms – the symptoms of symptoms – inasmuch as she feels the indignity of her primary symptoms. This partly recalls Jake's perceived social restrictions, although Liz's sense of indignity, as Anne MacLeod describes it to us, has an immediacy to it (that is, an emotional immediacy) that seems more present to her, more visceral in itself, than just the indirect recognition of social constriction, however painful that would be, either for her or, in his own circumstances, for Jake. The feelings of humiliation suffered by Jake of course might approach this.

Liz, too, looks beyond her symptoms in a predictive sense. Rather like Jake's self-imposed loneliness (even monasticism, until that decision is taken away from him), and in a more conscious and articulated echo of Rachel's habit of hiding herself and her compensatory drinking, Liz's knowledge of her disease and what it can do to her alters the way she lives her life. In effect, the epilepsy produces a different way of being Liz – what I shall later go on to suggest that we think of as a disturbance in her daily music, a clear form of discordance or dys-tone. She exhibits this different way of being herself quite consciously, in her dissembling as a way of coping with her situation – she had 'been lying for so long', she herself recognises ironically. As with Rachel and Jake, her own symptoms are obviously intrinsically unpleasant as well as being obstructive. Moreover, for Liz their sign-ness seems transparent.

In the case of the more elderly Jen and her stroke-ridden husband Geoff, there are on the face of it two sets of symptoms, one per sufferer, although it's possible that some of the deficits produced by Geoff's condition might make some of his symptoms less obvious to him. If so, then perhaps the essentially first-person nature of symptoms means that in Geoff's case their status and character as symptoms are to that extent diminished. We are not here concerned to explore Geoff as a fifth patient in his own right, because his patienthood is – or produces, or intensifies – part of the complex of Jen's own suffering, magnifying the consequences of any limitation that disease might place upon her ability to care for, and cope with, her husband.

Furthermore, if Geoff's symptoms are to some extent masked from him by the intellectual effects of his stroke, by contrast Jen is all too painfully aware of her own symptoms. Again, like Liz, she also has what we might call 'meta-symptoms' – symptoms of symptoms – the physical dizziness and faintness that assail her on realising what may be in store. We are all familiar with the physicality of perceived threats, the physical form that anxiety takes in response to those seemingly mental constructions, suspicion, doubt, belief, or even certainty with regard to a perilous future. 'I am faint when I think of the worst that they may do to me', confides Sir Thomas More, Robert Bolt's eponymous *Man for All Seasons*.[1] He might well speak for Jen, her knees loosened by what we might call the *institutional* signs – or even the institutional symptoms – of disease, the dreaded letter containing the hospital appointment, itself a symbol and sign of what is to come.

Allow me now to return to a sixth patient, one not intended or suspected when I initially met our first five, but one who, perhaps forgivably, for a while occupied my attention to their exclusion.

WHAT PAIN MIGHT MEAN

I am prey to every conceivable minor ache of muscle, tendon, joint. In concert they become a sort of scale-model of the agony of the rack, or of those mediaeval cages that deny their victims room to straighten up in any direction. No position of my limbs prevents their being locked in painful muscular tension; if I can muster the concentration and the resolve (and this is tiring in itself) I succeed briefly in releasing localised muscular tension only to be flooded anew by the aching of the associated joints.

However, this aching is nothing more than the backdrop to something more surprising and frightening, the far less familiar pain of profound coughing. In daily life, a cough is something you occasionally *do*, consciously perhaps, to clear your throat or relieve some tickling inner discomfort; you pay no attention to it, unless to defer it to a convenient time (the gaps in a programme of music at a concert) or to apologise to others for disturbing them (in a reading room or a library). The cough I now experience is no 'daily use' cough, and it is anything but voluntary – an internal tearing, ripping, pulling-apart pain significant enough to make me dread the next bout, especially if it assails me on being just roused from drifting off into a little sleep. The outrageous pain of coughing seems unopposed: I have no resources of preparation, pacing, bracing to fall back on. Why in pity's name should a cough hurt so much?

Now I rush to the bathroom to spit into the wash hand-basin. I idly notice that the colour of the expectorate has changed from yesterday's malevolent orange to a sullen ochre; is this an improvement? Over the coming days I will watch this ochre fade into salty transparency, though without noticing any great improvement in how I feel.

Right now the cough hurts so much that any concerns with what it might mean increasingly evaporate in the face of the more powerful concern that I simply not cough any more in that agonising way. The question of what the pain might mean is of course important, but it will have to wait: right now it's a question to which I just can't attend. My whole being is concentrated on simply not coughing, or – when that fails – on simply staying intact (I can put it no other way) through the next spasm.

THE 'SILENCE OF THE ORGANS'?

In exploring a distinction – such as that between a forward-looking bodily symptom that is also a sign to the sufferer, and a presently compelling symptom whose severity means that it consists simply in being suffered – it is often useful to draw on an analogy to help us. I am going to attempt a musical analogy, both because it occurs naturally to me as a musician, and also because it is invited by what is one of the most symptom-centred accounts of health and illness, namely that given some years ago by Leriche: 'Health is life lived in the silence of the organs.'[2]

For Leriche, the silence of the organs appears to consist in the absence of symptoms, and hence it seems that health consists in life lived in the absence of symptoms. (Leriche is well aware that this is not the same thing as the absence of underlying disease, but – controversially, no doubt – he seems to see the reality of disease as consisting primarily in its effects on the sufferer.) When this bodily silence is disrupted by symptoms, we both suffer those symptoms and also ask ourselves what they mean in terms of the present – and perhaps future – loss of our health.

This sounds like an attractively simple account of health. It, too, rests on an analogy with the world of sound. However, the analogy is itself too simple. In particular, it seems, we should assume that silence is an inherently good thing, the necessary background to whatever life consists in, and, in that context, wholly beneficial. However, to judge how helpful is this bodily analogy with silence, we need to think about whether silence *is* always a good thing, and we need to think about what silence makes possible – what life lived in bodily silence consists in.

The first of these considerations actually illuminates the distinction that chiefly interests me here – that is, between symptoms as such and symptoms which are also signs. Thus silence can be thought of as good in two senses – first, the direct and 'presently aware' sense in which silence is good just because it is the absence of disturbance (and disturbance is something we would almost always wish to avoid in itself), and second, the indirect and forward-looking sense in which silence is good simply because 'no news is good news': it does not threaten any specific future harms. When I am well, my bodily silence is both indirectly good in that it is not threatening, and it is directly (or intrinsically) good in that it is not unpleasant (not disturbing, distressing or jarring). The idea of silence as intrinsically good is distinguished by the contrast with those forms of sound that are intrinsically bad – sounds which are unwanted and intrusive, for the most part (although not exclusively) what we would ordinarily call noise.

However, it is also pretty clear that silence need not always be benevolent. Silence can in different contexts be itself threatening (the motor fails to start), disturbing (the normal hum of activity in your home street is suddenly absent), intimidating (a one-sided and uncomfortable conversation 'hangs' in the air), bizarre (someone misses their lines in a play or their entry in a musical ensemble), coercive (the parent refuses to acknowledge the child's apology and plea for forgiveness), manipulative (an acquaintance 'blanks' you in front of mutual friends), and so on. Even in bodily terms – the terms that interest Leriche – there is something odd about *not* feeling, for instance, that one is distinctly full after eating a very large supper, or *not* sensing the reassuring throb of tired muscles after a work-out in the gym or a long walk in the hills.

Even so, let us grant Leriche what he plainly intends here, that the silence of the organs is one in which they do not *intrude upon* our self-experience or self-awareness. What we might often think of as silence is, after all, only a relative matter. The silence in the cathedral prior to the start of the concert is of course not silence at all. The bored and reluctant concert-goer would pick up all kinds of stray sounds, but so long as none of them is too loud or abrupt, the eager concert-goer is still able to settle into a state of musical expectation and anticipation such that the distant crisp patter of tiny sounds accumulated in a huge vaulted space is still, effectively, functionally silence so far as the music is concerned.

Similarly, in ordinary experience the occasional passing twinges in a muscle, the rumbling tummy, the temporary feeling of being over-full, transient light-headedness on getting up too quickly, are all things of which we are minimally aware and we are happy to forget them almost at once – they do not constitute those sorts of intrusions (upon our sense of bodily self) that we cannot ignore.

It is in this context that the symptom is both a form of noise – something intrinsically unwanted now because it is intrusive – and also a sign, the articulated sound of something approaching. Bodily noise in this sense starts out as a symptom. When later reported, it may go on to provide meaning for the clinician, refined from the randomness of noise as such to something more directed – what we might call dys-tone or discord rather than mere noise; sounds with pathological meaning for the properly attuned ear. (For example, the symptoms of fever as an experience are also the signs of fever as an inflammatory response.) Up to a point there is a kind of interior dialectic between sign and symptom, for the patient and doctor communicating closely together. However, this depends on the extent of shared understanding. What is discordant or dystonic for the observing clinician may turn out to be very different from what is discordant or dystonic for the sufferer.

But in any case we are getting ahead of ourselves. The clinician hasn't come in yet – we are still (for this present volume) at the lonelier stage of the emerging, the 'dawning', of symptoms upon the incipient patient's awareness. And this 'dawning' is the awareness of a change, an emergence, an intrusion. We detect noise both by contrast with silence, and sometimes by contrast with tone. Both can scythe through our consciousness.

(Quite apart from the wholly voluntary evils of the mobile phone ring tone, the truly unforgivable cough at the concert is the one that breaks in upon the exquisite dying notes of the slow movement, and not the one that interrupts the prolonged silence between movements. I have personally seen someone ejected from a recital for sneezing in the 'overhang' of the final chord of the middle movement of Rodriguez' guitar concerto.)

It seems true that we need not be aware of silence except retrospectively. Compare the written silences in musical or dramatic performance, programmed and choreographed. The silence of bodily organs is not like this. It is more like the relative quiet of a sheltered suburban street prior to the rushing through of an emergency vehicle's siren – we only notice it when we've lost it. The silence is barely listened to while it yet persists, but it is mourned for what it was once it has been shattered.

Silence then has different forms, and it stands in contrast to different forms of sound – perhaps, as we shall see, different forms of unwanted sound.

LISTENING FROM PRISON

Being ill is, in part, being in a prison of uncoordinated, acutely perceived sounds – sounds made arbitrarily by others who are free to roam in a way that mocks the bedridden. I hear the characteristic sounds of lessening darkness – endless night though it seemed – the (to me) bewildering daily enthusiasm of waking birds. As the light grows, I can hear the first aeroplane out of the local airport; its passengers are today not one but two worlds away from me.

The sounds themselves might be particular to individual cases, but as a general phenomenon they recall something familiar to us all, the remembered illnesses from childhood which always seemed to consist in being obliged to remain in bed during the daytime, unwillingly (yet compulsively) listening to the ordinary and familiar noises of daily life being made strange and disconnected by being muted, heard as though from behind two or more intervening doors, the humiliating sounds of *other* children playing outside, out-of-doors, a place of mocking freedom that is for the time being constitutionally denied to the sick child. These sounds proclaim the absolute *miserableness* of everything when you are unwell, and refresh the inward protest against having to breathe nothing but 'indoors' for many days.

Right now such recollections are interlaced with the guilty but entirely unhelpful acknowledgement that these banal miseries are as nothing – *absolutely nothing* – compared to what is faced by those in for a long hospital stay, or genuinely bedridden or housebound. (How much better should that make me feel?)

SYMPTOMS, NOISE AND DISCORD

Noise stands in contrast to silence, but it also stands in contrast to meaningful sound, sound that has sense, purpose, direction – sounds such as music, for example. As we have noted, silence is one thing when it is the absence of mere noise, and quite another thing when it is the absence of meaningful sound or *tone*.

Which of these is 'the silence of the organs'? It seems to me that it can be either and both, and that ill health can correspondingly consist in simple noise but also in dys-tone or discord. Recognising this requires, I think, a more complicated account of that healthy life that is lived in 'the silence of the organs.'

The life that consists in doing what I want to do, or (which may not be entirely the same thing) living as I want to live, has direction, purpose, rhythm and structure. To me as a musician, the analogy of health as life lived consonantly with its own form of music is one that arises naturally. When illness interrupts this it produces – what? Noise? Or discord, where this is more than (for the musician, sometimes worse than) noise? It depends on the forms that the symptoms take, and on their severity.

Leriche himself seems to suggest something like this in his claim: 'That which produces disease in us touches life's ordinary resiliences so subtly that their responses are less that of a physiology gone wrong than that of a new physiology where many things, tuned in a new key, have unusual resonance.'[3] It seems to me that this intriguing suggestion is true in some symptomatic states of ill health but not in all of them, and when it is true it is so only to an extent. Those symptoms that merely obstruct my living as I want to live (for instance, fatigue, weakness, stiffness) are, I think, best considered as noise, impeding my usual access to the familiar music of my life. By contrast, those symptoms that disrupt my conscious experience of the world, those symptoms whose intrinsic awfulness 'un-makes' my ordinary experience of the world,[4] produce in its stead a twisted experience for as long as they last, a new and bitter music to which I am forced to listen. As Canguilhem expresses it from the point of view of physiology: 'Diseases are new ways of life.'[5]

Indeed they are, and not for physiology alone. Simple noise obstructs my access to music, whereas discord replaces concordant sounds with a twisted version of those sounds. We can 'turn off our attention' from noise far more readily than we can suppress our awareness of dys-tone, dysphonia, twisted music. In music as such, we tolerate or actively enjoy a certain amount of discord within manageable limits (these limits obviously vary for different individual listeners, not to mention composers). However, in health and sickness the tolerance of discord is far, far lower, and individual variations in our tolerance of bodily discord are viewed with suspicion, or even 'pathologised' (for instance, as masochism or as attention-seeking behaviour). Perhaps this shows another limitation upon drawing the musical analogy strictly, but it is no more than a limitation. The essential distinction between what I am calling 'instrumentally unwanted' symptoms and 'intrinsically unwanted' symptoms seems to me to be upheld and illuminated by it. Beyond mere noise, 'intrinsically unwanted' symptoms replace not only the silence of the organs, but also life's familiar music with active discord. They command my attention, they oblige me to turn my gaze inwards upon itself involuntarily, inwards upon a different and unwanted, unpleasant, perhaps awful way of being me.

LIFE AS MUSIC, INTERRUPTED

So instead of adopting Leriche's conception of health as life lived in the *silence* of the organs, I would like to suggest a notion of health as life lived in the quietly concordant *tone* of the organs – concordant one with another and with the facts and circumstances of our daily life. Health is life lived in the ordinary music of our daily experience. This music depends, certainly, upon a background of reasonable silence – life presently unthreatened, unencumbered by my state of being. If either the music or its supporting silence is interrupted by too much noise, too many obstructive symptoms, then I will be prevented from doing what I want to do. But if either the music or its supportive background of silence is interrupted by discord, as I have characterised it here, then while *those* symptoms last I am forcibly diverted into an intrinsically wretched, damaged, painful way of being in proportion to the severity of the symptoms. Discord in this sense is not noise but rather *tone made hideous*. Its grip befouls our ordinary attention, making it hard to notice or respond to life's ordinary music. (Indeed some discord is so severe as to amount to unfiltered cacophony beneath which life's ordinary music is obliterated. Heath describes the overwhelming effect of prolonged acute nausea, while suffering from paralytic ileus, as both focal and unbearable, irresistibly commanding hideous attention.[6] We want only that the pain or the nausea or the suffocating breathlessness should stop; we long for silence before ever again we can contemplate music.)

WHAT IS IT TO RECOVER?

When we are genuinely labouring under the symptoms, all we want is health for its own sake, intrinsic health, health that is the silence of the organs – not even, as Leriche thought, *life lived* in the silence of the organs. We want *simply the silence*.

But it is all so transient, and we patients so fickle. Show me but a hint of recovered function – turn down the volume on but a single one of these hateful things – and old possibilities once again re-present themselves to me. Perhaps after all I will get back to the treats and treadmills of my ordinary life. Turn down the symptomatic volume generally, leave me at least sitting up and taking notice, and the instrumentality of health towards my other ends and goals, rather than its intrinsic goodness, is what I remember.

What is it to recover? That sense of the body's decline – has it a mirror on the upward slope? Do we (as said a friend after an appendicectomy) marvel to see our own organic systems coming back to life? Perhaps; although in comparison with the sheer hunger to 'be' authentically once again, I fear my own sense of marvelling would be brief on a scale familiar to quantum physics. Looking ahead to recovery from within illness's prison, my undoubted attitude would be one of greed, greed to get back on to the escalators, even the treadmills, of (to pinch, and adapt, a phrase of Fulford's[7]) ordinary doing.

ILLNESS, 'ORDINARY DOING', AND ORDINARY BEING

A more recent account of health and illness draws especial attention to the obstructive aspects of symptoms – in my own terms, the noise that gets between us and the music of ordinary life or, in the terms of the account's author, Fulford, the pathological obstacles to 'ordinary doing', the bodily deficits that lead to a failure of ordinary intentional action.[7]

Fulford's account has many virtues, and one of them is his restoration of illness to a position of primacy over disease, echoing Leriche in the process – it is because we fall ill that we seek medical help, and the medical categories of disease arise in an attempt to understand, explain and respond to illness. Individual cases of illness may arise because there are diseases, but conceptually, as a classification of our knowledge of the world, the category of diseases is there because we are prone to falling ill, and because we have an interest in knowing how best to deal with our predicament.

However, in stressing 'ordinary doing' as the coinage of health, Fulford emphasises an action-centred view of life and of the self, reflecting a widespread conception of ourselves as above all *agents*, reflected elsewhere in the age of technological achievement and restless endeavour – for instance, in morality, where most approaches to understanding and forming moral judgement focus on action and agency, emphasising the question 'What should I *do*?'. It is in conspicuous contrast to this that virtue ethics, probably alone among mainstream western moral theories, asks instead 'How should I live?', 'How should I *be*?'

The two aspects of symptoms that I have been trying to distinguish in this chapter reflect this contrast. Those symptoms that constitute noise are those which impede action – they impede 'ordinary doing.' They are instrumentally unwanted, they get in the way, they signpost future obstacles to action, perhaps worse. They also confirm an instrumental view of health, emphasising what health is for, in terms of the things that we can undertake and achieve when we are healthy.

However, those symptoms which twist our ordinary experience and make it bitter do not so much impede what we want to do as divert us into a wretched way of *being*. They confirm an essentially intrinsic view of health, reminding us that sometimes we want nothing more than to feel better, to feel as we ordinarily feel, to regain silence as much as proper tone.

Much is sometimes made of the idea that as patients we can invest illness and symptoms with meaning and understanding, and thereby lessen the suffering. But it seems to me that it need not always be like this. The possibility of meaning might intensify the suffering. In the end what I want is to be able to be myself in a way that I understand and am familiar with. Beyond this, but only when I'm restored to it, I can think again of the projects I want to complete, the actions I want to undertake. The propensity of symptoms to impede us sometimes stands aside in favour of their propensity to overwhelm us. Perhaps when I am well, my idea of being well is embedded in acting and doing, but when I am sufficiently ill, all of this matters less than just being able to *be* well again, simply to *be* the breathing, sensing, creature who, freed from pain or nausea or the fight for breath, can once again look around, outward and inward, and remember what it is to be me.

REFERENCES

1 Bolt R. *A Man for All Seasons*. New York: Vintage Books; 1960 (this edition published in 1990).
2 Leriche R, quoted in Canguilhem G. *On the Normal and the Pathological* (translated by CR Fawcett). New York: Zone Books; 1991. p. 91.
3 Leriche R, quoted in Canguilhem G, op. cit., p. 97.
4 Compare with Scarry E. *The Body in Pain: the making and unmaking of the world*. Oxford: Oxford University Press; 1985.
5 Leriche R, quoted in Canguilhem G, op. cit., p. 100.
6 Heath I, 2006, personal communication.
7 Fulford KWM. *Moral Theory and Medical Practice*. Cambridge: Cambridge University Press; 1990.

CHAPTER 2

The body as lived experience in health and disease

CARL-EDVARD RUDEBECK

'EXISTENTIAL ANATOMY': THE SONG OF THE SELF

Time

The body constitutes the self physically, and is the bearer of its existence. No body, no self. Experience is brought about instant by instant. One experiences nothing of shorter duration than an instant. The Germanic languages use *Augenblick* – the time it takes the eye to see something, which implies the time it takes to perceive the world anew. The instant is thus both the shortest unit of lived time, and the smallest unit of experience. Time is living and it is given through the senses, both through their incredible sensitivity and imagination, and through their limitations.

One's body measures time through its rhythms – heartbeats, breathing, thirst, hunger, the emptying of bladder and bowel, sleeping and menstruation. The rhythms are links to the unknown body, and that which is beyond conscious control, but so long as they keep their expected patterns, they bring about security. One rests on the rhythms of the body.

The longest experienced time is one's own life, one's age. Beyond these limits, time disappears into infinity.

One's age implies statistics – what, on average, could be expected in terms of outlook and capabilities given a certain sex and age – and it is the person, naked before the mirror. Often their own age surprises people, but in fact they do not know what they are surprised about.

Movement and space

Through the movements of the body, the relationships between the self and the social and physical world change. Movements in context are actions. There are definite limits to the freedom of movement. Gravity ties the body to the earth. Freedom of movement is greatest when gravity works within the self in a natural way. Thus freedom of movement is constituted as a certain relation to its restrictions, which is demonstrated beautifully by the little child, sitting totally relaxed with straight back, playing on the floor.

With the risk of suffocation at a safe distance, breathing is a wave-like rhythm in the body, the optional and the imperative relying upon each other. Hyperventilation is an escape from the imperative, while striving for the control of every breath is mistrust in the optional. Both are losses of spontaneity.

The self is at the origin of the world. Far away, close to, above, underneath – all of these have the self as their point of reference. Being is a dimension of space. The archive standard metre in Paris is as much an agreement as it is exact. Movements turned into experience disclose space as meaning. To become space it has to be inhabited. One cannot be in front of the house, and at the back of it, at the same time. In order to know that the surface outside the window is a house with a circumference, one's mind has to walk around it. Experience is space-time. The theory of relativity also makes sense in the life-world.

Man stands on two legs, his feet silent and hard-working, but sensitively establishing contact with the ground. Standing up provides us with an enlarged view and, at the same time, allows the self to be seen by others. The breathtaking moment of standing for the first time lives on deep inside. Standing and walking are independence. Falling is a threat. Running is hunting and being hunted, but is also playing. As they get older, most people stop running. Life is running on and away.

The trunk of the body connects the head and the limbs. It holds the self together. It belongs to walking and standing and is at the centre of grips and gestures. The intentions spread through the body from this vulnerable centre. Keeping in touch with the vulnerable is part of bodily harmony.

The trunk is the slave of the self, the back that bends under heavy burdens.

With the arms one tries to reach the world, while the touch of the hands has the potential to change it. In manoeuvres such as gripping, banging and digging, the hands complete the work of the arms. In delicate work it is the reverse. Here the hand is the head of the arm with movements that have the intelligence of a brain. The things touched, and the tools used, relate to the self through the functioning of the hands and arms. Until one interacts with it in a concrete sense, one remains a stranger in the world. The piece of wood in one's hand is no less part of the world than the tree from which it was once cut out.

Hands are relations to others – from the soldier's salute of subjection to the intimate touch between lovers. Gestures are the capital letters of spoken language.

The head, too, is part of the body, but this may almost be forgotten when seeing an expressive face, and sensing the spirit within a gaze. However, sometimes it is the fifth limb, used by an African woman carrying a huge burden, or by a football player heading a ball whose impact might have knocked other people out. The head is also closeness to the brain. One can almost hear the sound of intense thinking. Although consciousness includes the entirety of a particular moment, and thoughts may be about anything, thinking itself is felt in the head. Whether this feeling is directly given, or is experienced by inference from knowledge, is hard to say.

In *existential* anatomy, the head is, above all, mind. Being that, it is more than any other part of the body the bearer of the vulnerability of the self.

The senses

The ear listens, which is one's way of being in the moment of listening. The world becomes sounds, silence, and directions encompassing the listener. Person and attention are one. Music takes the ear beyond the horizon of sounds. It is the language of the ear, as immediate as the vibration of the eardrum, as the stirring of emotions. The ear is also hearing in the semantic sense – that is, our being among other people who understand each other, naming our common world. When nothing is understood, we have exclusion. Yet, standing on an ancient piazza, listening to the murmur of many voices and languages, one may feel at home again irrespective of location.

The eye sees. It puts the world 'out there' with its gradations of light and shade. Seeing is light which always evokes the sun. Like flowers we turn our faces towards it. Light springs out of darkness.

Not seeing, one is within that which is not seen. Not hearing, one is outside that which is not heard. Deafness is more of exclusion from the world than is blindness. Seeing is understanding. It may not be possible to see the totally unknown. It is easier to put the known into it, to misunderstand in an informed way – 'I see.' What is seen reflects all that has been seen before throughout life. There is always recognition in discovery.

In its scientific sense, medicine is also an eye, undressing the sufferer in the cool of instruments and observation. His unknown future is the characteristic of his situation as a patient, but this same unknown is the province of the doctor's authority, and hence the grounding of the doctor's self-esteem. The eyes are surprise and disbelief. However, rubbing them does not remove the unbelievable from the stage of reality.

The skin is appearance, that which others see. Few regard their wrinkles as signs of experience. The skin is a protective boundary, and it is nakedness. It is contact with others and the longing to be touched. It is contact with the world – wind, water, heat, cold. The skin of the hand sees the familiar objects of a dark room. The skin is also a setting, a stage, for embodied emotions. The blush of embarrassment is itself embarrassing.

The nose smells. Smells are silent and invisible messages from the world, and from the past. They are atmosphere, and enhance or blight experience almost like emotions. In a pleasant room one may feel the presence of wood, spices, flowers or other things that one's nose likes to trace or remember. A bad smell cannot be distinguished from the nausea that it provokes.

The nose is quiet breathing. When congested with a cold it carries the feeling that there is not enough air. Breathing through the mouth makes public the hunger for air. Someone may disapprove.

Outdoor smells open up the landscape – the smell of pine trees in a northern forest, of steaming fertiliser over the fields, of cold itself on a clear winter day. Personal smells signal the closeness of a relationship.

The mouth opens to swallow the world, the same world to which it itself belongs – testing, enjoying or craving. Thirst arises discretely in the drying membranes of the mouth, and all of a sudden can turn into a longing for drinking, a drive stronger than anything else.

At the back of the mouth, swallowing meets breathing. On the level of the vocal cords, thoughts become embodied – become body – and then, through the pharynx, tongue and lips, communication. One's immediate radius of impact on the world far exceeds the dimensions of the body.

In a kiss, one gives up bodily boundaries. Closeness is taste, bodies embrace mucous membranes.

Sex

In common

Sex is a bodily fact that chooses one's name, and that comes before hetero- or homosexuality. It is not easy to know what in the self comes from one's biological sex, and what belongs to the role that one and others have chosen. The body is freedom and it is destiny. Sexuality is sex as a mode of existence. It is always there, even when it is not expressed.

Sex is a form within the body. It is there in every part as a resonance of the organs that actually define the body as female or male, and that embody love and reproduction.

For the woman

Menstruation and fertility define the three stages of female biological life – before, within and after. Time is inscribed on to the woman's body.

The womb is everyday bodily inwardness with toilet visits and daily care. It is also the form of relation to another – her lover – a longing for fullness colouring the world of senses. Within intercourse, pleasure is relating, and relating is pleasure, and both are body.

The womb is sensitivity. Are things the way they should be? Menstruation is the link with inner sex – regular, adding month to months, and reminding. Even if nothing else would change, change is there.

The breasts are sex, but they are also just breasts. Sensuality and concreteness alternate. In moments of pleasure, the whole body is pleasure. The breasts are also the sucking lips of the feeding baby, and the peaceful little face. It is thus even for an older woman.

The breasts are vulnerability when they lie flattened for the mammography camera.

In pregnancy, the child enters into the life of the mother as an experience of something still unreal, in which love grows unnoticed. Soon enough, however, the child climbs over the edge of awareness, becoming weight and movements. The big belly points in the direction of delivery. There is no escape. Forces will work, pain may be overwhelming, and there will be the baby. Will it be all right?

For the man

Where the woman has two biological transitions, the man has one. He has no other periods apart from the moon and the calendar.

His penis and scrotum are everyday bodily inwardness with toilet visits and daily care. They are also the form of relation to another – his lover – a stiffening longing colouring the world of the senses. Within intercourse, pleasure is relating and relating is pleasure, and both are body. His sex is his strength as well as his fear of exposing weakness, which here, in front of the woman, is the most concrete of exposures. The man's sex is mainly on the surface. The life of the prostate is silent. In the era of tests for prostate-specific antigen, it may seem to promise nothing more than cancer, and the weak urinary flow of old age.

The inner organs

The interior of the body is peace, with gusts of unrest in the dark. Warmth is generated. With listening senses one turns inwards but does not reach much further than to the rumbling of the stomach. Right there is the edge of the abyss, and questions thrown out from it get no other answers than the body itself. Requests for meaning should not be addressed to one's physical depths. If any answer comes, it is about meaninglessness.

The heart

The heart beats in the chest, in the depth of the body but still vulnerably close to the surface. One feels its steady rhythm – it is life, no more, no less, that moves in there. In excitement and strain, the heart takes over the whole chest, almost the whole body.

The heart is the heart of will and decisions, and the sensible target of critical remarks. It bears the emotions that withstand the reasonable – love heats, grief aches, happiness jumps, fear squeezes.

The heart divides the time given to each one of us. One of those beats will be the last. That is impossible to deny, yet it often is denied.

The emotions

Emotions are bodily experiences with their meanings in the world. Their variations unfold somewhere between the lump in the throat and the butterflies in the stomach. One may watch them from behind one's own face. This inborn mirror is the tool for practising disguise and self-control.

Emotion is a relationship between the self and its conditions. It is a certain mood sounding in the body, and it is never totally missing. Where emotions are lacking, the lack is itself the emotion.

Within the body, emotions are both similar and distinct. They are all variations of each other. Tingling is both longing and worry. Very deep emotions tend to hurt, irrespective of what they are about.

Emotion has its location in the body, but it is, at the same time, the whole character. Grief is heavy, making the steps slow and the head bend down. Joy is ethereal, the feet barely touching the ground.

Emotion is pace. There is the quick, jumping joy, but also idle and slow moods, when oneself is a good place to be in. Although one thinks of grief as slow, it can also be hectic, an escape from silenced weeping.

An emotion is the pitch of a certain moment, in which world and self sing the songs of each other. The song of the self is, without distinction, body and thought. Meaning arises as contact between the two. Like whirls, mere patterns of movement, it has no substance of its own. It is all about change. Different emotions are similar. Boundaries are drawn only in what is written down.

BEING, BODY, AND THE WHOLE OF EXPERIENCE

Existential anatomy is the body as it is experienced through all the passages of life.[1] Life's situations are not primarily about the body, but about the self and the world, and it is the body that ties the two together. The body is the form of relating to another, and it is sensuality. It is the unfolding of the real, itself included. When detached from its context, the body stands out as essentially concrete. It is fat or thin, tall or short, youthful or ancient, male or female. It bleeds when it is wounded, breaks when it has fallen from sufficient heights. It loses its subjective and existential role.

Beyond the surface of the visible body, a spectacular physical reality has been laid out, and the discovery of the body is continuously extending into its minute details, like an infinite microcosm.

Optimism accompanies this worldwide venture. Finding the answers to the most intriguing and crucial questions of human life is thought by many to be, more or less, a matter of time. Materialists even look forward to the scientific and concrete discovery of the mind, wiping out the distinction between the mental act and the observable correlates of that same act. However, it is hard to envisage that the activity seen on a PET scan will ever give access to the experience and meanings of consciousness itself, even though one is there, in the world, through a body, which it is possible both to observe and to manipulate by technical means.

Most of the time, we do not worry much about this fact. So long as things are as usual, which means that not too much noise is perceived from within the body, one's attention remains oriented mostly outwards in physical and social space, and forward in time. One is at home in the body. The energy and capabilities are there, as is the ability to enjoy the body. The recognition of being vulnerable is transformed most of the time into a reasonable and barely conscious level of taking care. Hence, normality is not about a neutral level between the positive and the negative. It is in itself positive. It is feeling alive in a 'homelike' way.[2]

Experience is perception, affect and cognition giving birth to an active and moving bodily subject, instant by instant, throughout life. There is always sensing, always an affective tone, and always a semantic structure. Any of the three may dominate at a certain point in time, and we name the corresponding mental act accordingly, but none of them is ever pure.

At every instant, what is experienced is a whole. There is usually a dominating focus of attention, while other aspects of the experience reside in the background. This foreground/background form of the whole of experience is the experiential and theoretical basis of gestalt psychology and gestalt therapy.[3] The degree of attention paid to the various aspects of the whole depends on the meaning of the experience. Moments of experience succeed each other without interruption through shifts of attention. Every moment in one's life is the instant idea of reality. Perception and interpretation run concomitantly. There is not first a perceived reality, and then the act of giving that reality meaning. Meaning is primordial to humans. In Gadamer's hermeneutics, the being of man is about understanding.[4] Even meaninglessness has meaning as meaninglessness. Consciousness is always directed towards something – either externally, or inwardly (introspectively). This is what the phenomenologists mean when they say that consciousness is intentional. The logical and challenging implication of the gestalt psychologists' recognition of the whole experience of a certain moment is that, whatever is perceived, more than that is perceived. There is no such thing as pure body experience, or pure attention to somebody else, however open and intense the latter may be.

In experience, the body is usually the background, presumed or tacit, of the perceptual field – 'the dark in the theatre', as the French phenomenologist Merleau-Ponty put it.[5] One does not see the eye that sees. However, in contrast to the view of writers such as Sartre[6] and Leder,[7] the body is neither completely 'surpassed' nor 'absent.' The background of experience is not emptiness. It is the self, alive in the body, spectator and creator at the same time. Bodily presence is more than the sudden itch on one's back disturbing a mind operating in splendid isolation. Self is always also self-as-body. Nor is the body fully an object among objects when it is observed by the self. It is always 'with me',[8] and one cannot turn it around to get a better view, nor can one move around it. The hand is not a distinct object resting on the table beside pencils and sheets of papers. It is part of the permanence of the self which, along with all the other parts, is 'integrated in a peculiar way; not spread side by side but enveloped in each other.' Although it is seen from outside, it is experienced from within, as an aspect of the self that is ready to handle things.

So the body that in everyday thought and talk seems to be straightforward and easily grasped is, when attended to closely, quite ambiguous. One's only access to it is existential. The self lives it. The body is always the self, but not only that. It is an aspect of the physically given world, but not only that. Here, at the interface of two contingencies, the body emerges as lived body. More clarity should not be expected. The symptom descriptions of medical textbooks are based on observation, and aim to present typical clinical pictures for recognition, while the patient's much less rigid account expresses experience and individuality. To avoid confusion and frustration, neither of these two versions, each valid in its own context, should be forced upon the other.

The body has its place in any situation that could possibly be experienced. There it has its form, either withdrawn, as when one relates to somebody or something, or in focus, such as in moments of self-absorption. Those parts of the body that happen to be within the visual field are just one aspect of the body experience. However, although what is seen is very incomplete, it is essential to the completeness of the experience. The visualised body has its distinct boundary, while the lived body has its transitional zones or horizons of intentionality, where it emerges as meaning – self as body or 'my body'. In its outward intentionality – the 'ecstatic body' in Leder's vocabulary[9] – it relates to the world. Inwardly, it rests on the body as biology and nature, and is exposed to nature's implacability. Only in those two relationships is it possible for a person to put into words what the body is about. The semantic field that is unfolded here *is* the 'existential' anatomy.

Outward intentionality is primarily about participation in the world. Life has a practical character. One is out there, relating to the world through the senses, and with the size, mobility, speed, strength and robustness of one's body. The body is that of which one is capable under the conditions given. Its form is its possible and executed actions, and thus it is tool-like.[10]

Inward intentionality is, most of the time, like a discrete but permanent scanning of the background of experience. To give priority to what is given externally, one cannot be preoccupied with the body. The interactions with the world therefore bear the silent message that the background is indeed as much 'in the background' as it should be and, therefore, health probably prevails. When, to take the opposite case, unequivocal signals from within the body claim attention, the world itself becomes background. The sensations may be either discomfort or bodily pleasure.[11] It is their distinctness that matters.

The pictures on the pages of descriptive anatomy textbooks show a transparent, often skinless order. Everything is in place, layer by layer, and organ by organ. Even the dermatologist looks *through* the patient despite having the patient's skin as the subject of specialisation. When the medical gaze focuses upon a certain and peculiar patch of the skin, the patient's existence is of limited interest. During the diagnostic phase, giving information when asked to do so may be the maximum communication allowed to the patient. This cannot be held generally wrong, since every situation has its optimum mode of verbal exchange, but any doctor needs to be continuously alert to the reductive power of the clinical setting. Even the patient may be chasing the machine within the body. However, in the beginning there was experience.

Here the symptom once stood out from the background of the existential anatomy.

THE SYMPTOM: WHAT IT IS

Semantics

In the original sense of the word, a symptom is a change in a person's physical or mental condition, due to disease. It is the task and power of medicine to decide whether or not a certain experience is a symptom. However, there is significant slippage in the meaning of the concept. When a general practitioner talks about 'symptoms presented in primary care', or meditates over the very low predictive value of those symptoms, he or she refers to experiences that *might* be due to disease. Epidemiology has contributed to this conversion of a causal relationship between disease and symptom into a hypothetical one between symptom and disease. Here it is the character of the experiences, rather than their potential significance, that matters. The implication is mainly experiential. Symptoms are about illness. They are those bodily experiences that intrude on life, and are perceived to be abnormal. Still, the causal sense of the concept 'symptom' lies parallel to the experiential one, and thus when discussing symptoms one might refer to anything from a very specific disease symptom to a fleeting sensation in a sensitive person. It is therefore wise to try to make the reference explicit. Although the symptoms described in Anne MacLeod's stories are mainly 'real' symptoms, in this chapter the perspective is more that of an open situation when the patient first visits the doctor. In certain passages the connotation will be more specific, but that will be made clear.

A change or difference

The most general feature of a symptom is that it is a change of, or difference in, self-perception that is perceived by the subject not to be normal. In this volume, the emphasis is on bodily symptoms, but of course the difference may equally well be within the emotional–cognitive domain. The separation of these two categories of symptoms is an abstraction in relation to experience. Experience is always perception and affect and cognition. Nevertheless, symptoms are mainly about one or the other, or about the transition between the two. People define this fairly distinctly themselves – body, soul or stress.

Change is prominent in new symptoms. It turns into difference when the abnormal becomes the individually normal, as in diseases that may not be cured or balanced.

Change is what happens to Rachel. Very little is as it was before. Since change is gradual, she is fighting fiercely to adapt, but she seems to lose herself in her awful predicament. It is so totally dominating as to make her feel that it has no beginning and no end. She is falling out of time – the most dramatic of changes, outrunning the very meaning of change, since being out of time means having no references. It is free falling. At the stage when we meet Rachel, it would not matter much if she were a grown-up woman. Earlier in the development of the disease, however, change would then have provoked reflection and protective measures, after an initial period of surprise and hesitation. The child lives change all the way through, while the adult sees herself cast out by it, and therefore strives to come back to the normal.

Jake's skin is *difference*. He is difference. He perhaps does not even remember when change burst upon him. His immediate impulse, very naturally, is to hide. Then his skin becomes loneliness and the fear of being seen which, at the same time, is what he wants most of all. He wants to be touched, and yet what he then imagines is the dry sound of hyperkeratosis caressed, and his skin in flakes on the body of a woman, and on the sheets.

Liz's difference is hidden. It is an unreliability implanted in the midst of herself. The organ of consciousness is rebelling like a volcano, and therefore the integrity of her mind is put in question. Suddenly she will find herself helpless in a supine position anywhere in the world, her mind trying to hold onto that world through the heavy haze of the dissolving fit, slowly noticing the moisture and smell of stools and urine, and having no escape whatsoever. Her difference also has its place in culture since the origin of culture. Modernity has not wiped it out. The difference consists as much in others and their judgements as in herself. She is her difference, and she is not.

Something permanent

Usually experience is a continuous shift of situations. The self-as-body is at the centre, making the situation up, however discretely, from the conditions given by perceived reality. Most of the time, attention is out there. Perceptions in the body tell more about the situation than they do about the body. The heartbeat dwells within jogging and feeling cold within an icy wind. When the situation comes to an end, so does the part played in it by the self-as-body. The permanence of the self-as-body, necessary for being somebody, is its intentional horizons, not that which emerges at those horizons. When a symptom takes its form within consciousness, it is not only a change – change is the norm – but something that breaks out from the constant variability of experience as a certain permanence or rigidity.[6] It need not be there all the time, but must be recurrent enough to become something in itself – a new phenomenon within the self-as-body. It is a serial story in consciousness, and through its permanence, it has a life and identity. However, to discern the symptom as something, the self has to be something to itself. The child bears the symptom innocently. The alien is not questioned. It is just another, but more troublesome, way of being.

With stubborn permanence the bloodied cough is pursuing Jen. Many times she has stood by the basin, hoping that this time the awful red colour will not appear. But no, there is something she simply cannot pass by. It has to be faced. And outside the bathroom door her husband stands waiting for her, as if he knows that the warning sign which he has never seen also involves him, thus giving family medicine a sad but significant implication.

Permanence is what maintains the difference. Liz is an epileptic even in the long intervals when she is free from fits, and she needs medication. Permanence means ambivalence about taking medication. It helps, but it keeps her difference close to her and, taking the lid off the container, she hears her mother's anxious voice and 15 years just disappear.

A rift in that which is taken for granted

A symptom is not just a dab of discomfort on the unchanged remainder of daily life, but a streak of helplessness and unease in the whole, and sometimes much more than that. When one passes from 'everything is perfectly all right' to 'something is wrong', the body stands in the way of itself. The change does not need to be dramatic. It is a rift in that which is taken for granted, the rift that causes the trouble. The body no longer feels at home, otherwise it would just have been one experience in the endless sequence of experiences. It is this rift that makes symptoms ranging from the trivial to the ominous belong to the same category of human experience.

Contingency

In the experience of one's own body, much is passing just at the fringe of attention. What is made conscious is very contingent. Well-known perceptions step forward more easily but may also pass more easily, so long as they confirm 'homelikeness.' However, those that signal a possible threat tend to linger, and to become enhanced. This contingency is the soil in which symptoms grow – the same sensation in physiological terms may send very different messages to an individual, depending on the circumstances. Different people pick up and interpret sensations in different ways. Not until the bodily derangement is considerable does experience mirror in a more or less unequivocal fashion the situation of the body.

In the stories of Rachel, Jake, Liz and Jen, the margin of negotiation between the self and the body as nature is small. Their diseases break through into the field of intersubjective recognition, into the public arena. To them, the body and its functions are an obtrusive fact.

THE CONTEXT OF THE SYMPTOM

Something is wrong in the body

When something is wrong in the body, it will show sooner or later. An experience will emerge that is impossible to refute. The body-as-nature displays its physical autonomy. It attracts the attention of the subject, who tries to understand and to get to grips with the situation. There is a continuing inward vigilance, and thus the experience gets its form also in time. When the symptom is intense, it catches our full attention, and our contact with the world and with others becomes seriously weakened. The intentionality of the primarily bodily symptom is *introverted*.[1] The degree of introversion is a measure of the seriousness of the condition. Rachel even locks the door against an outside world that she cannot endure any more. Introversion is loneliness, and it is meaninglessness, since the body is hardly relating the self to others any more. It is implosive. Jake's introversion is more complex. It is running away both from the eyes of others, and from the insistent presence of his own skin, the latter demandingly distracting him from his relationships.

Introversion may work in more protracted and less obvious ways. When a deadly disease at a certain point reaches the decisive change and becomes dying, this may be understood at some level by the ill person[12] as a knowing from within the body. The irreversible course of life, which everybody knows in the abstract, becomes concrete. Time is the fading of one's own body. One's pain is also the pain of the loss of the world. Jen, losing weight and coughing blood, is probably approaching the situation where death is presence rather than absence.

In introversion that is caused by a symptom, the inner horizon of the self-as-body becomes the focus of attention. The experience is taken over by the body-as-nature. This is a body 'other than me.'[4] The self has very little control over its functions, and most of them are beyond the inner horizon, and thus beyond awareness. It stands out as an immediate fact, presenting one's existence and then making it complicated.

A symptom that is primarily of a bodily character therefore brings two messages. The first is about the specific features of the condition – location, degree of damage, possible cause, and so on. The second is about vulnerability in general. Death is just beneath the surface of many consultations. Correspondingly, a patient has two requests when presenting a symptom. The first is 'Help me' and the second is 'See me.' This sequence is not necessarily anything to do with importance, but is rather to do with the ease with which these requests are brought up with the doctor. There is reason to believe that the second one is often dealt with *en passant*, between the lines of explicit communication. To Rachel, helping and seeing are the same. Where she is right now, existence amounts to biology. Morality and the use of technology walk hand in hand, which is the ideal situation of biomedicine. To the other three individuals pictured by Anne MacLeod, both requests have to be taken care of separately.

Something is wrong in life: the situation

Experiencing oneself is, at the same time, experiencing one's situation, and experiencing a situation is always, to some degree, experiencing oneself. Where the emphasis should lie – on oneself or on the surrounding world – depends on the circumstances. Situations put their imprints on the individuals concerned. The burdens of life have their absolute weight, but this is experienced differently in different situations. Burdens belong to life. In carrying the burden, one may say that the burden is carrying the experience. Strain and friction are inherent in life.

At a certain limit, drawn very individually, a strain becomes troubling. The variations are due to differences in strength and endurance, and to differences of perception, which are in turn dependent on the implications of the strain in question. Pain that, whatever its present origin, opens the wounds of embodied traumatic experiences easily becomes unbearable.[13] Withstanding the pain of prolonged strain is, at the opposite end of the spectrum, an important element in the talent of a cross-country skier. Unless he reaches the stage of pain, he will not succeed.

Most discomforts that refer to demanding situations never develop into symptoms. As experiences they are too obvious to raise suspicions of disease, or too fleeting to give the hope that medicine would have anything to offer. However, beyond the limits of tolerance, discomfort becomes suffering, or worry, or both, and then the doctor may become a refuge. The difference between this suffering, and a suffering that comes namelessly from within the body itself, is that the meaning of the first is within the situation. It expresses a relation to the world, and as such it is more 'extroverted' (that is, outward-facing) than introverted. Fatigue and pain in the shoulders may reveal the situation on the factory production line, and sudden and recurring pain in the stomach may indicate that something extremely irritating is going on. The 'extroverted' symptom is coloured by emotions, the bodily element of which is quite often the complaint. Grief is the lump in the throat. The emotion is not the cause of the symptom but rather the symptom itself. In this situation the very physical aspect of the symptom, despite the attention it receives, belongs mainly in the background. Otherwise the symptom would not have been extroverted. The doctor senses the symptom's intentionality when it fills the room. He is brought into the relationship. The situation is very different from an introverted presentation, where the body-as-nature talks in a fairly low voice. Here the symptom may even remain hidden behind the veils of confusion or fear.

Inattention or denial may blur the context of the symptom. Introversion and the suspicion of disease then tend to take over. Certainly when the meaning of the symptom is hard to accept, it may be obscured by a conviction that it is of basically bodily origin, and thus a case for medicine. It acquires a weight that makes it even more 'extroverted', since the symptom presentation also becomes an appeal for the recognition of the suffering, and of its presumed causality.

Ambiguity

When they are long-standing or extreme, stress and strain may actually damage the body. What begins as a temporary and conditional situation in the body becomes a derangement, with an ensuing impairment of function. It becomes complicated to sort the situation out, since the release from the probable overload will not give relief from the symptom, which is now characterised by a physical life of its own. However, with regard to its intentionality, the symptom is indeed *ambiguous*, because limiting the therapy to the biologically conceived body, the body-as-nature, will not give permanent relief either. A certain degree of ambiguity often accompanies many extroverted symptoms, depending on how distinctly the body-as-nature steps out from its background position. Jake's irritable bowel indicates a certain bodily disposition. Other people just become nervous in situations of anxiety or stress, and still others react with different symptoms. Even introverted symptoms may have a streak of ambiguity. When a person has become accustomed to a disease and, with it, a given level of function, attention then tends to be directed mainly outwards towards the world, when new discomforts appear. Possible and substantial limitations of capability may be overlooked or underestimated by both patient and doctor in common optimism.

Rachel is suffering from a severe somatic disease, but she does not yet know it. Her family interprets her behaviour in context, which is usually where interpretation begins. Most 10-year-old girls do not get diabetes. The misunderstanding adds seriously to her loneliness – it is a very sad story – and at the same time increases her exposure to physical risk. This kind of error of judgement is very much feared by the medical profession, quite under-standably. However, the fear seems to be sublimated by the profession into a norm, as a result of which the extroverted symptoms become but a diminutive anomaly and remainder after the real diagnostic work has been done. Here, the evident is lost. If the doctor looks at nothing but the mucosa of Jake's bowel, Jake will be left alone in his predicament, and the investigation will also be incomplete. Sensing the intentionality of symptoms should be a crucial clinical skill.

EXISTENTIAL TYPOLOGIES OF SYMPTOMS

'Existential' anatomy gives the symptoms their accurate bodily implication. Clearly extroverted symptoms are almost all existential anatomy. The meaning and the symptom are synonymous. Tension headache is tension, but still it aches. Sensations from the body-as-nature provide the substrate that becomes meaning within the right context, and the stronger they are, the more they crave attention in their own right. This 'pure' physical dimension, whether it is the substrate of the extroverted symptom, or a primarily biological impairment, has its specific features in the middle of action or experience. There is no pure, detached, bodily reality, and therefore disease is not just disease. Everything is lived. With the disease or derangement, the conditions of life change. Some symptoms are in a concrete sense the loss of a capability, others are more an obstacle to entertaining a capability that basically is there, while still others represent the invasion of the self-as-body by the body-as-nature through discomfort, suffering or worry, or the direct impact on consciousness. Mixtures of these main typologies of symptoms often occur. At the same time, once they are there, symptoms change the relationships to others, and to the world, depending on their specific features. The original character of a symptom is most distinct when it first appears. The longer it has lasted, the more it is modulated by emotions and thoughts, and the more it becomes part of the experience of the body as a whole, where yet other symptoms may live. In the long run it may even lose its meaning as symptom and step into the background of an ever developing normality.

Losing a capability

Jen's husband, Geoff, stroke-ridden as he is, may experience an unconditional loss within consciousness itself. If this happens, thoughts halt before their conclusions, and memories often become no more than shadows, mocking in their incompleteness. He may be aware, in a strange way, of those fading areas of awareness that formerly were recognition of the world, feeling and reasoning. The limits of his inner life are the painful demonstrations of the grounding of the subjective in the biology of the brain (i.e. in nature). No one knows whether his anxiety and bad temper are the 'true' interior of his personality coming into the open, or the despair from saying farewell to those subtle qualities of mind that formerly really were him. If the latter is the case, all he may hope for would be the succeeding loss of the neurons bearing the insight into and the darkness of his predicament.

Serious mental losses caused by tissue damage in the brain are quite understandably, but still paradoxically, caught through observation rather than through the accounts of the experience of loss itself. The very meaning of losing aspects of cognitive and emotional life dissolves into the vagueness of expression. Emptiness in this very definite sense is a real challenge to empathy. It is not easy to imagine that which simply is not.

Loss of motor function impairs the interaction with the world in very concrete ways. If one prepares the movement to seize a slice of bread on the kitchen table, and then suddenly finds that the arm just does not lift – it is as if it were not there at all – a provoking emptiness finds its place in the middle of one's body. The hand is nothing but an unfinished act. Helplessness is what is left of the original intention to have a slice of bread. The agony and puzzlement of losing a limb that is physically present has been described by Oliver Sacks in his book *A Leg to Stand On*.[14]

Losing functions is part of the life cycle. The fading of the singing of crickets during the summer nights symbolises ageing. One listens, but all that remains is the dark, turning memories into loneliness.

The symptoms of loss restrict the interaction with the world in a way that is implacable, so long as the symptom lasts. The body-as-nature is now absence. When it was working it was not attended to, but when it is absent, everything changes. With persistence of the symptom, accepting it becomes a process that in fact is a change in self-perception.

Being hindered

When bodily changes hinder psychomotor capabilities that are themselves in fact intact, the body traps itself. The capability is preserved inside the restrictions caused by stiffness, pain, hoarseness, weakness, breathlessness or other symptoms. In concrete terms, however, life may become empty or strained. One may, temporarily or permanently, have to retire from the activities that are most enjoyed, or the most important, but the capability is close, and there is no absolute emptiness within the certain field of the existential anatomy. In the permanent situation, acceptance is about respecting the frustration and anger as a path towards patience, and from there to make the best out of the changed conditions.

Evidently, 'trapping' symptoms are very common, but it happens that none of the patients in Anne MacLeod's stories suffers from a fracture, from arthritis or arthrosis, from cardiac or respiratory failure, or from any of those diseases that most saliently go with that kind of symptom. Jake, however, is socially trapped by his physical condition. He sees himself with the eyes of imagined others, and finds himself quite disgusting. He limits his social interactions to situations that are safe, and here he also has to take his irritable bowel into consideration. He leads a life below his potential, but as the story highlights, his situation is conditional, although his psoriasis is a fact. There are very few things that he really cannot do, or that he has to refrain from doing, and the eyes of the real others – the colleague at the hotel, and Carol – see a person very much worth relating to. What we may learn from Jake, with regard to diseases that imply more definite restrictions, is that there is no absolute relationship between the factual symptom and its gross consequences. Other individuals might have been less afflicted, or even more greatly afflicted, by the same skin disease, and the implication of, for instance, distal arthrosis in the hands – ailment or catastrophe – depends on the role of one's fingers in one's life project.

Being invaded

To some extent, physical symptoms are always invading one's experienced normality. However, some symptoms are more clearly intrusive than others. Their main effect is a preoccupation of mind, and a corresponding distraction from attention to the world and to others. Capabilities are not specifically affected. Itching and irritation, pain, coughing and worry are forceful invaders even when the disease itself might be quite benign. Infections yield the model for the invasion metaphor, and other military metaphors in medicine as well, and with generalised symptoms, biology and experience here walk hand in hand. From one day to another, a bad cold may really determine one's whole existence. In life-threatening disease, vitality itself is invaded by physical destruction, reducing existence to blank biology.

The sense of invasion is first and foremost linked to the debut or increase of a symptom. It is dynamic, and its reference is former experience. Accepting the symptom as a fact makes it easier both to deal with it, and to judge it. Conversely, denying the emerging state of nature within one's own body adds a drama to the original one. If the symptom then persists, the situation will be chronically acute, hindering the assimilation of the symptom and the adoption of a new idea of normality.

In Rachel's case, the very normal sensation of thirst turns into an invasion, since it breaks through without reason – strong, and impossible to satisfy. The well known is at the same time totally alien, yet Rachel takes responsibility for being invaded, hiding her enormous intake of soft drinks and water. There is a very basic shame in being fully nature, and as such being out of control.

Jen looks at the blood in her phlegm. She has seen her own blood many times, but now it is the wrong time and place, and that gives her a strong feeling that something is there that should not be there. Fear increases the invasive power of the probable serious disease, and she is pulled away from her home and her husband into an inner and frightening place. It takes effort to cling to the daily practicalities, and she may feel that all there is left of her attention is a facade.

For many years Liz has been living with the constant threat of having her awareness overrun by epileptic fits. Her self-image is therefore always slightly invaded. The closest she gets to the very experience of invasion is the aura and the post-fit confusion and emptiness. When the fit is there, she is not aware of it herself. Although caused by neurophysiological deflection, in experience the invader is another and uncontrolled form of existing, apparent only to those who stand by. Their fear and helplessness help us to understand old notions that the gods were involved, punishing the person, or even inhabiting the body in convulsions.

THE PERSONAL AND THE GENERAL

The medical conditions of Rachel, Jake, Liz and Jen expose them all to their bodies-as-nature. They are forced to live that which healthy people often push aside but, beyond the individualities of their diseases, they mark the existential baseline of all humans – vulnerable, mortal, and with a physical construction of great conformity, even though the differences are often more attended to. At the same time, one's body is closer than close. It is intimacy and shyness. Thus it is both the most general and the most private in life. The symptom experience, packed and conveyed in the symptom presentation, has an 'I' and an 'it', but the 'it' is no less human and moving than the 'I.' Medicine acts precisely at this ambiguity. Its knowledge aims at the general, its practice tumbles into the private and existential, and therefore its ethics has to discover this practice, over and over again. Here is the energy of the medical encounter.

REFERENCES

1 Rudebeck CE. Grasping the existential anatomy – the role of bodily empathy in clinical communication. In: Toombs SK, editor. *Handbook of Phenomenology and Medicine.* Dordrecht: Kluwer Academic Publishers; 2001.

2 Here Svenaeus refers, through its negation, to the term 'Unheimlichkeit' introduced by the German phenomenologist Heidegger to give the character of 'the ill forms of life.' In Svenaeus' vocabulary and understanding, homelikeness is health. See Svenaeus F. *The Hermeneutics of Medicine and the Phenomenology of Health: Steps towards a philosophy of health practice.* Linköping: Studies in Art and Sciences – Department of Health and Society; 2000.

3 Perls F, Hefferline RF, Goodman P. *Gestalt Therapy. Excitement and growth in the human personality.* Harmondsworth: Penguin Books; 1973 (first published in 1951).

4 Palmer RE. Hermeneutics. In: *Gadamer's Dialectical Hermeneutics.* Evanston, IL: NorthWestern University Press; 1969. pp. 194–217.

5 Merleau-Ponty M. *Phenomenology of Perception.* London: Routledge & Kegan Paul; 1962.

6 Sartre JP. *Being and Nothingness. An essay on phenomenological ontology.* London: Routledge; 1956.

7 Leder D. *The Absent Body.* Chicago: Chicago University Press; 1990.

8 Merleau-Ponty M, op. cit. p. 90.

9 Leder D, op. cit.

10 See note 2.

11 Toombs SK. *The Meaning of Illness. A phenomenological account of the different perspectives of the physician patient and patient.* Dordrecht: Kluwer Academic Publishers; 1992.

12 Feigenberg SG. *Terminal Care. Friendship contracts with dying patients.* New York: Brunner/Mazel; 1980.

13 Kirkengen AL. *Inscribed Bodies: health impact of childhood sexual abuse.* Dordrecht: Kluwer Academic Press; 2001.

14 Sacks O. *A Leg to Stand On.* New York: Touchstone; 1998.

CHAPTER 3

Issues of privacy and intimacy at the beginnings of illness

IONA HEATH

> I was all right on the Monday. I was all right on the Tuesday. And I was all
> right on the Wednesday until lunchtime, at which point all my nice little
> routine went out of the window.[1]

Alan Bennett's Miss Schofield, *A Woman of No Importance*, struggles to understand the beginnings of the stomach cancer which is to end her life, to make
sense of her experience by pinpointing the first intimations of illness. From
a distance of more than 30 years, I recall a similar account. I was a newly
qualified doctor, I was clerking the morning's admissions and I was in a
hurry. I was listening to an old man – or at least I thought of him as old then,
but I fear that he may have been no older than I am now. He had suffered a
myocardial infarction at about 11 o'clock that morning and he was telling me,
in minute detail, about when he had got up and what he had had for breakfast.
I now understand that he was trying to give me all the clues that might explain
why this catastrophe had struck him at this particular moment. He wanted me
to understand his situation before his illness had begun, because he thought
that this would help to throw useful light on his current predicament. The
problem was that, fresh from my medical education, I thought that I already
knew all there was to know about myocardial infarctions and, to my shame, I
could barely conceal my impatience.

An enormous amount has happened before a patient tells his or her story.
How do we, as we become sick, identify and acknowledge the very beginnings
of illness, those first inklings that something is not right somewhere in the
body or mind – the first whisper of pain, or the first suggestion of a swelling

or a rash, or the first glimpse of an unexpected trace of blood? How do we communicate these first hints to ourselves and then to others? All of these processes are profoundly affected by issues of privacy and intimacy.

FEAR AND SENSIBILITY

In his essay on Modigliani, John Berger writes:

> Everything begins with the skin, the flesh, the surface of that body, the envelope of that soul. . . . And everything is completed there too. Along that outline are assembled the stakes of Modigliani's art.[2]

It is also along that outline that the stakes of illness, of medicine and of clinical relationships are assembled. Illnesses begin within the outline of the body. They may be induced from without, but they begin within. Gradually or suddenly, our attention is withdrawn from our quotidian engagement in the world and is relocated inwards to examine the minute workings of body or mind.[3] The body, usually so taken for granted, draws attention to itself in a manner which is more or less difficult to resist. Sometimes the beginnings are so gradual and insidious that they can go unnoticed for years; at other times they impose themselves immediately and forcefully on the consciousness of even the most distracted or stoical. A dying friend, a man, once told me that he thought that the requisite inward perceptions were more acute in women than in men because they were honed more regularly through the experiences of menstruation and pregnancy. As a generalisation, this seems unlikely to hold, but it does seem probable that individuals are more or less sensitive to their bodily environment, just as their ears and eyes are more or less discriminating.

> Every human being is probably born with a natural bodiness which, if allowed to develop, is characterised by balance, coordination, and awareness of space. Like any genetic gift, this one has been differentially distributed. Those who live more intensely in their own bodies than others probably have a certain richness of nuance in the flow of impulses from within their own body. Depending on their other personality traits, this may of course be either a great advantage or a source of persistent torment.[4]

For everyone, a major driver of bodily sensitivity is the existential fear of suffering and death which continually impels and heightens vigilance. Persistent torment seems most likely in those unfortunate enough to combine insecurity and fearfulness with this heightened inward sensibility. Most young children like Rachel are relatively immune to existential fear but, as we grow older, we become increasingly aware of the inevitable finitude of existence and ever expectant of the first inexorable signs.

TS Eliot touches on the growing inevitability of fear in his play *Family Reunion*:

> When I was young and strong, and sun and light unsought for
> And the night unfeared and the day expected
> And clocks could be trusted, tomorrow assured
> And time would not stop in the dark![5]

BEGINNINGS

The moment when feelings are first articulated into thoughts of illness and thereby privately acknowledged as symptoms is the beginning of an illness story, which can be short or long.

> Slowly the Truth Dawns
> To waken, and feel
> your heart sink
> heavy and dark
> and hardening . . .
> Slowly the sea lifts its billow,
> slowly the forest reddens its gorge,
> slowly the flames begin to lick in hell,
> slowly the truth dawns.[6]

Olav Hauge's poem provides an astonishingly precise description of a sensation hardening into a symptom, a fear crystallising and becoming explicit.

Context and circumstances can either facilitate or inhibit the acknowledgement of feelings as symptoms. In recurring episodic illnesses such as Jake's irritable bowel syndrome or Liz's epilepsy, familiarity may spur acknowledgement, but it may also, perversely, be so intrusive and disruptive of ordinary life that it breeds denial. Similarly, fear promotes acceptance, but within fear lurks another fear, which is that of appearing foolish if the original fear proves unfounded, and this second fear works in the opposite direction. Different individuals are more or less able to dismiss and repress their fears. Jen's story shows how easily the earliest symptoms can be pushed aside in the face of the burdens, stresses and responsibilities of daily life.

Similarly, different individuals are more or less capable of putting the needs and concerns of others above their own. Geoff, in the face of his disabling illness, cannot do this, but Jen still can. The experience and story of the life before the symptom, and the context within which it appears, dictate much of each individual's response to it.

> Time present and time past
> Are both perhaps present in time future,
> And time future contained in time past.[7]

The interweaving of past, present and future has a powerful effect on the manner and speed with which feelings become thoughts and perceptions become symptoms. What happened when I felt this sensation before? Did I feel foolish or relieved when it resolved – or both? Do the feelings seem similar to those described by my mother or father at the beginning of a serious illness? Has my closest friend been given a life-threatening diagnosis in recent months? Am I looking forward to some particularly important occasion which could be threatened by this new feeling?

Space and place can also both either inhibit or facilitate. Where am I when I become ill? How safe is introspection at that moment and in that place? Yi-Fu Tuan has written about the difference between place and space – the former providing the fixity necessary for security, and the latter the opportunity for movement and exploration.[8] From the safety and stability of a known place, each of us is aware of the openness, freedom and threat of space, and vice versa. Place offers the possibility of privacy; space is more often public. The perception of both is affected by the onset of illness, often with a heightened sense of the security of the one and the threat of the other, so that place can allow the acknowledgement of symptoms, while space may prevent it.

Each of us, aided and abetted by a variable combination of sensibility, preoccupation, fear, denial and stoicism, sets the boundary between the significant and the insignificant at a different point. Each of us allows a feeling to become a symptom at a different threshold.

HIERARCHIES OF NEARNESS

The most near to me is myself. Within the isolated individual, where is the locus of control?[9] Who is risk averse and who is not? How much fear or uncertainty can each of us hold alone – and for how long? How have our life stories, our culture and our context made us as we are?

– panic mounts up easily in the chaotic and depleted space inside him.[10]

The immediate family is usually next in the hierarchy of nearness and, at this point, privacy gives way to intimacy:

– privacy and its special gift which is intimacy.[10]

Privacy shared is intimacy, but families are more or less intimate and help or inhibit the expression of illness to a very variable extent. What are the family stories? What is told and not told, shown and not shown? Which are the bonds of trust? Who notices distress, withdrawal or preoccupation in others? Who notices pallor or pain or loss of weight? Who feels responsibility for whom? Who can and cannot be told? Who can and cannot hold and contain their anxiety about themselves or each other? Who must not be troubled or burdened?

Jake has moved away from his family of origin, and is not yet secure enough within his developing relationship with Carol. Liz is trying not to burden her young child with the reality of her illness, and Rachel is inhibited by her fear of being told off. Geoff's preoccupation with his own predicament effectively silences Jen.

Beyond the family, what context is provided by the neighbourhood and community? Are relationships close and possibly intrusive, or distant and indifferent? Both families and communities may have strong traditions of stoicism or symptomatology. Some individuals, families and communities, perhaps particularly in areas with a long history of heavy manual labour, have a tradition of independence, austerity and fortitude which values self-reliance, and which may lead to a significant delay in allowing illness to become explicit.[11] Similarly, some family histories encourage a sense of fatalism and an expectation that health will begin to deteriorate at a relatively young age, and this too may lead to a slowness to complain and to pass on complaint.[12] Other communities and other families do exactly the reverse.

Beyond immediate neighbourhoods and communities, there are public stories, which are read every day in the newspapers and heard on radio and television.

In every situation except the most everyday, most neutral ones, a pressure is exerted as to how we should behave, how we are to feel. And when one looks at the matter a little more closely, one discovers not infrequently that novels, films and theatre pieces which one has seen or read somewhere have dictated these roles for us.

> When reality confronts us with unusual situations, we first reach for these emotional stereotypes common to novels.
>
> They don't give us much footing. They make us lonelier than before, and head over heels we fall out into reality.[13]

How and to what extent do these public stories influence the perception and disclosure of symptoms?

Despite the ever wider dissemination and availability of such public stories, the extent to which different individuals are exposed to or sheltered from them remains highly variable. This in turn may lead some individuals to adopt illness stories that are familiar from hospital soap operas with a minimum of adaptation, while others, deprived of such templates, must struggle to construct a more authentic account.

For those suffering psychosis, the impact of public stories is more direct, and characters and actions from television and radio may be incorporated directly into the personal narrative of the individual, causing both confusion and distress.

Doctors and other healthcare professionals have a place in the hierarchy of nearness which can fall anywhere, depending on the particular patient, the particular professional, and the nature of the relationship between them. It seems likely that Jen feels much nearer to the doctor than Jake does. For some, the doctor is the very first person to be told, while for others they are almost the last, and all the same factors apply. How open and attentive is the doctor? How much uncertainty and fear can the doctor tolerate? How much risk is there in appearing foolish within the particular relationship? How much does the doctor notice?

WORDS

When privacy moves to intimacy, thoughts must become words in order to be shared. What happens? What are the processes by which feelings become thoughts and thoughts become words? Each stage seems to require compression and reduction as the experiential is constrained within the linguistic. Thought lags behind feeling[14] and words lag behind thought. How much is lost and to what extent, if at all, is it possible to recover what is lost?

Subjective experience and the feelings that it invokes are free-floating and infinite, yet completely unique to the individual. Concretised into thoughts, feelings begin to be both structured and restricted. The next step by which thoughts are further concretised into language imposes another layer of structure and restriction.[15] Experience, feelings and thoughts are necessarily lonely, and only when expressed in language can they be shared. Precisely because they are shared, words represent what is universal in human experience.

Mikhail Bakhtin described the way in which words are changed and refracted by each usage – continually subject to both centripetal and centrifugal forces.[16] As each one of us appropriates words for our own purposes, we add our own particular shade of meaning, producing a centrifugal force which continually develops and fragments language. Yet at the same time, all language is social and built on the attempt to achieve shared and centripetal understanding. The words spoken by those who are sick are the closest we can come to the human experience of illness. They represent only a shadow of the totality of that experience, but they express the most that we are able, through language, to share.

Once articulated, the power of words to make us feel less alone is astonishing and consoling. They are both the means and the ends of the human compulsion to search for meaning. They form the map which outlines our understanding and, at the same time, guides our search for more. Words help us to make sense of our daily experience of joy and suffering, and make it absolutely clear that those experiences are shared, at least partially, and that, to this extent, we are less alone.

However, as soon as thoughts are expressed as words, they become public and there is the possibility of embarrassment and of appearing foolish. Symptoms are driven by fear, but if the fear turns out to be groundless, one may feel foolish. Intimate relationships enable embarrassment to be risked in a way that public relationships do not, which is why the relationship between doctor and patient, although formal, must remain intimate.

> Men and women . . . have words. With their words they change everything, and nothing. Whatever the circumstances, words add and take away. Either spoken words or ones heard in the head. They are always incongruous, because they never fit. This is why words cause pain and why they offer salvation.[17]

And expressing the same contradiction:

> Words can cause trouble like large rocks in one's path.Wrong: Words can clear the largest rocks out of the way.Wrong again: Words can turn into dark chasms unbridgeable for a whole lifetime. We know very little about the power and the destructiveness of words.[10]

Meaning is inevitably changed during the movement from private to public, from inner to outer. The challenge for the listener is to minimise that change and to approach as closely as possible to the inner, private experience. And having listened, the next daunting challenge is to find words to contain what we have heard and to demonstrate and communicate our understanding.

It is more and more common for those who feel ill to use medical words such as 'palpitations' or 'depression' without fully understanding what these words convey, and this can serve more to conceal than to reveal the true nature of the subjective experience.[18] When this happens, the listener may need to gently reject words or phrases which have become formulaic, and attempt to come closer to the original experience.

Some people make it very hard for us to listen, let alone understand:

> His only weapon was abuse, the rebellion of the helpless – without hope but precisely because of that, deserving admiration and respect.[19]

And there is no doubt that admiration and respect provide at least a starting point for listening. Rachel's petulance hints at her helplessness but, at that moment, those around her are distracted by other things and no one is listening or able to recognise what is happening.

> This individual and closely intimate recognition.[20]

There is a need to come close enough to see and to hear, and so to recognise, but there is also a need to provide space so that both speaker and listener have room for manoeuvre. It is a dialectic of closeness and distance, with the latter emphasising an imperative of respect that guards against a premature, invasive understanding of the other. This oscillation between closeness and distance is also that between empathy and analysis, and it has to be held and concentrated in what Henry James described as 'the palpable present intimate.'[21] The present moment is the moment of speaking and the moment of listening:

> All meaning, understanding, and interpretation is inherently negotiable and tentative. Likewise, there are no fixed meanings transferred in conversation. All participants in a conversation bring with them totally different worlds, and are continually shaping these worlds in the process of dialogue. This reshaping requires the intimacy of conversation – that we remain in continuing language contact with each other.[22]

The dialectic of closeness and distance and indeed the whole fluid nature of conversation resist the dangers of a pre-emptive certainty.

The listener, whose immediate reaction and response can have a profound and lasting effect on the outcome, carries a huge but mostly unexamined responsibility. Through our attitudes to each other, we shape each other's worlds, for better or worse.[23]

PRIVACY IN PUBLIC

Most illnesses begin in the private inner world of the suffering individual, and will only be revealed when and where there is an offer of intimacy. However, there are some illnesses which abolish privacy at their very beginning, and the situation becomes one of 'privacy in public'.[24] Getz and Kirkengen used this phrase in relation to women's experience of pregnancy, but it also describes many other situations, including accidents, sudden disabling or embarrassing illnesses such as Jake's irritable bowel syndrome, fits such as those provoked by Liz's epilepsy, and other visible problems such as rashes and palsies. As soon as Rachel's collapse or Liz's fit is discovered, their earlier privacy immediately becomes public. Although this must have been Liz's experience, she still struggles to maintain her privacy and, in so doing, emphasises its fundamental importance.

DENIAL

Denial and its companion virtue, stoicism, seem always to have been part of the human response to illness:

> It is part of the balancing act of life that one learns to forget what is causing a disturbance, or at least succeeds in regarding it with indifference. One of the means for sustaining this skill of balancing is precisely intelligent behaviour, including, for example, self-deception or the knowing refusal to accept the truth of one's own illness.[25]

The more serious the illness, the more likely the sufferer is to deny something of its reality and so embrace this 'knowing refusal.' However, there is a striking disparity in the ways in which denial is interpreted in physical and mental illnesses. Denial is often regarded as courageous in the face of serious physical illness, but is usually found reprehensible in the mentally ill. Indeed, part of the stereotypical description of patients with mental illness is that they lack insight into their condition. Yet there is no obvious reason why someone suffering a disturbance in the mind should be less likely to seek to protect themselves through a form of denial than someone whose disordered functioning seems to be more firmly located in the body. Denial on the part of the sufferer may lead an observer to underestimate the severity of the condition, while a perceived lack of insight may have the opposite effect. Someone who has a serious physical illness and is also under enormous psychological and emotional stress may resort to a combination of denial and suppressed insight, creating a story which can be very difficult to interpret.

These confusions illustrate the extent to which illness reveals the artefactual uselessness of the traditional Cartesian mind–body split. Physical and mental distress are aspects of a unitary condition:

> A man's body and his mind, with the utmost reverence to both I speak it, are exactly like a jerkin, and a jerkin's lining; rumple the one, you rumple the other.[26]

However, when mental illness begins to predominate, issues of privacy and intimacy rapidly become problematic:

> The things I thought were real are shadows, and the real
> Are what I thought were private shadows. O that awful privacy
> Of the insane mind![5]

Despite much effort to address this, mental illness still carries a significant stigma, which means that privacy may be even more closely guarded. The pervasive, atavistic fear of madness and disintegration means that the apparently 'normal' can be very keen to draw a clear demarcation between themselves and those others who suffer mental illness. This can mean that opportunities for intimacy and the sharing of privacy are much more limited. Sufferers are, to a greater or lesser extent, excused their responsibilities within society, but are also systematically excluded, albeit in a way that is no longer as cruel as it once was, but that nonetheless often remains judgemental and condemnatory.

NÆR-GÆTNI

I discovered this wonderful Icelandic word[27] in the summer of 2005, and wonder how I had managed so long without it. It means 'near-carefulness' – the carefulness required by nearness. It is a deliberate condition of intimacy, and it is an essential precondition to the sharing of those intensely private feelings and thoughts which mark the beginnings of illness.

REFERENCES

1 Bennett A. A woman of no importance. In: *The Complete Talking Heads*. London: BBC Books; 2001 (first published in 1982).
2 Berger J. *The Sense of Sight*. New York: Vintage Books; 1985.
3 Toombs SK. *The Meaning of Illness. A phenomenological account of the different perspectives of the physician patient and patient*. Dordrecht: Kluwer Academic Publishers; 1992.
4 Rudebeck CE. General practice and the dialogue of clinical practice: on symptoms, symptom presentations and bodily empathy. *Scand J Prim Health Care*. 1992; **Suppl. 1**.
5 Eliot TS. *The Family Reunion*. Orlando, FL: Harcourt Brace & Company; 1939.
6 Hauge OH. *Leaf-Huts and Snow-Houses*. London: Anvil Press; 2003.
7 Eliot TS. Burnt Norton. In: *Four Quartets*. London: Faber and Faber; 1943.
8 Tuan Y-F. *Space and Place: the perspective of experience*. Minneapolis, MN: University of Minnesota Press; 2001.
9 Bosma H, van de Mheen HD, Mackenbach JP. Social class in childhood and general health in adulthood: questionnaire study of contribution of psychological attributes. *BMJ*. 1999; **318:** 18–22.
10 Berger J. *Photocopies*. New York: Pantheon Books; 1996.
11 Tod AM, Read C, Lacey A *et al*. Barriers to the uptake of services for coronary heart disease: qualitative study. *BMJ*. 2001; **323:** 214–17.
12 Richards HM, Reid ME, Watt GCM. Socio-economic variations in responses to chest pain: qualitative study. *BMJ*. 2002; **324:** 1308–11.
13 Gustafsson L. *The Death of a Beekeeper*. London: Collins Harvill; 1990.
14 Vetlesen AJ. Introducing an ethics of proximity. In: Jodalen H, Vetlesen AJ, editors. *Closeness: an ethics*. Oslo: Scandinavian University Press; 1997. p. 6.
15 Hastrup K, Hervik P, editors. *Social Experience and Anthropological Knowledge*. London: Routledge; 1994.
16 Bakhtin MM. *The Dialogic Imagination: four essays*. Austin, TX: University of Texas Press; 1981.
17 Berger J. *Lilac and Flag*. New York: Vintage Books; 1992.
18 Puustinen R. Voices to be heard – the many positions of a physician in Anton Chekhov's short story, A Case History. *J Med Ethics: Med Humanities*. 2000; **26:** 37–42.
19 Herbert Z. *The King of the Ants*. New York: The Ecco Press; 1999.
20 Berger J, Mohr J. *A Fortunate Man: the story of a country doctor*. Harmondsworth: Penguin Books; 1967.
21 Henry James. Letter to Sarah Orne Jewett, 1901.
22 Anderson H, Goolishian HA. Human systems as linguistic systems: preliminary and evolving ideas about the implications for clinical theory. *Family Process*. 1988; **27:** 371–93.
23 Løgstrup KE. On trust. In: Jodalen H, Vetlesen AJ, editors. *Closeness: an ethics*. Oslo: Scandinavian University Press; 1997. p. 79.
24 Getz L, Kirkengen AL. Ultrasound screening in pregnancy: advancing technology, soft markers for fetal chromosomal aberrations, and unacknowledged ethical dilemmas. *Soc Sci Med*. 2003; **56:** 2045–57.

25 Gadamer H-G. *The Enigma of Health: the art of healing in a scientific age.* Palo Alto, CA: Stanford University Press; 1996.

26 Sterne L. *Tristram Shandy.* 1759–1767.

27 I am grateful to Professor Vilhjálmur Árnason for the gift of this word.

CHAPTER 4

Vocabulary of health and illness: the possibilities and limitations of language

JOHN SAUNDERS

INTRODUCTION

The inmates of Hell were healthy: they needed to be. But we have become less interested in that, and since the Renaissance have a dwindling interest in an afterlife of perfect health.[1] The early experience of illness has come to interest us more, yet not as one of life's expected hardships, bestowing no special status or worthy of no special consideration. That beginning, that early experience, may result from our current obsessions with screening and the identification of risk factors. A middle-aged man walks into the doctor's consulting room, his blood pressure is measured, a middle-aged patient walks out. However, the commoner experience is still that of Rachel and Jake and Liz and Jen. We articulate our early experiences, initially in our inner conversation with ourselves, and later in our dialogue with others. We think or talk, not necessarily in that order; and we use words.

PEOPLE TALKING

It is the use of language that distinguishes us from other animals. Only human beings communicate with one another by a 'true' language – that is, by vocalisations that may have abstract meaning and which are subject to inflections and variations of syntax. Foraging bees reputedly convey the direction and distance of provender to their hive mates by means of stylised flight patterns and dances. This primitive communication develops as we climb the evolutionary ladder to the grunts and grimaces of the lower anthropoids. As Medawar and Medawar have observed,[2] language cannot have begun in the form it was said to have taken in the first recorded utterance of Lord Macaulay. After his hostess accidentally spilled hot tea on him, he first bawled his head off, but then, after calming down, responded to his hostess' concern by saying 'Thank you, madam, the agony is sensibly abated.'

Gua, the chimpanzee, was born in captivity and brought up alongside an Indiana couple's own baby.[3] The child performed slightly better in the serial intelligence tests during the first nine months. However, the advantage was small compared with the child's prospective intellectual superiority which was to become apparent. By responding to people who talk to it, the child soon begins to understand speech and to speak itself. By this one single trick in which it surpasses the animal, the child acquires the capacity for sustained thought and enters on the whole cultural heritage of its ancestors. This has been summed up in three points. First, the intellectual superiority of humans is almost entirely due to the use of language. But, secondly, the human gift of speech cannot itself be due to the use of language, and must therefore be due to pre-linguistic advantages. Yet, thirdly, if linguistic clues are excluded, humans are found to be only slightly better at solving the kind of problems we set for animals. The inarticulate faculties which produce speech are in themselves almost imperceptible. The use of language has tacit roots.[4] These opening observations lead us to reflect upon language and its use. This is not simply a matter of using it better, improving our grammar or syntax or vocabulary or pronunciation or accent or the intervals of silence. Rather it is to acknowledge its centrality in all that we say, to acknowledge the differences between a computer printout or a synthesised voice message on the railway station announcements compared with our groping for language to construct and express our experience as intimations of illness impress themselves upon us. The railway announcement tells us that the train is late, the talking clock tells us the time of day, the voice on the telephone tells us to press button 2 for a certain service. They communicate information. However, illness demands that we do rather more than this, and language has a wider variety of functions.

It would be hard to over-emphasise the importance of communication in medicine – in diagnosis, treatment, support and overall care. Its failures are constantly highlighted, its importance in curricula has increased, and its value is featured in all professional guidance. Here, for example, is the General Medical Council's view:[5]

Good communication between patients and doctors is essential to effective care and relationships of trust. Good communication involves:

➤ listening to patients and respecting their views and beliefs
➤ giving patients the information they ask for or need about their condition, its treatment and prognosis, in a way they can understand, including, for any drug you prescribe, information about any serious side-effects and, where appropriate, dosage
➤ sharing information with patients' partners, close relatives or carers, if they ask you to do so, having first obtained the patient's consent.

Language is what distinguishes doctors from veterinary surgeons. Doctors and human patients talk to each other: 'At the heart of the physician's practice is the consultation. The patient's history must be carefully elicited and recorded . . .'[6]

LANGUAGE'S FUNCTIONS

Following Crystal, let us set out seven functions of language.[7]

Emotional expression

The patient experiences pain and shouts an oath, or experiences relief from some symptom and cries out in relief or gratitude. No one else need be present. Nothing is necessarily communicated, for there may be no one there to communicate with.

'. . . that label. Epileptic,' says Liz to herself. The words or phrases that we use are commonly conventional enough, but can reach an occasional level of literary sophistication.

Social interaction

'Morning, Harry,' says Jen. Ritual exchanges such as 'Good morning', 'How do you do?' communicate nothing in the usual sense. We say 'Bless you' in response to a sneeze or 'Cheers' as we down a drink. Even the popular 'Have a nice day' usually indicates no real wish (although the London taxi driver's response of 'I'll bloody well have the sort of day *I* want,' does provide an occasional contradiction).

Power of sound

Rhythmical litanies of religious groups, dialogue chants by slaves and prisoners, or the language games of children as they play are examples. 'I like coffee, I like tea, I like radio, and TV . . .' as the ball is bounced off the wall or the ground. Other examples are the unintelligible sounds used in songs (ging gang gooly, doopey doo, hey nonny nonny) or the glossolalia of the religious.

Control of reality

Prayers, invocations and formulae directed at God, gods, spirits, objects or other physical forces are a highly distinctive form of language. The response is appreciated only in the mind of the speaker, or there may be no evident response at all. 'How could such a slip of paper seem so heavy?' protests Jen.

In the healthcare setting, such speech is often silent yet probably almost universal, even being used by the most sceptical. Atheists bargain with God in their heads. Language becomes the vehicle for aspirations which seem tardy, uncertain or impossible of delivery.

Recording the facts

This function is represented by all kinds of records – data banks, case notes, scientific reports, and so on. The facts are stored for possible future use, but may never be referred to again. Our hospitals are full of this. Nothing may be communicated, as it may never be read.

An expression of identity

The chanting of slogans at public meetings, the shouts of affirmation at religious meetings, and the stage-managed responses of an audience in a television game show inform us of little. Such chanting fosters the solidarity between those who share the same view or participate in the same occasion.

The instrument of thought

We often speak our thoughts aloud. We hold conversations with ourselves or we calculate arithmetic aloud. Language enables complex thought. We can express ourselves with gesture or pantomime, but both suffer when internal speech is disturbed. Finger language and lip-reading, as practised by deaf mutes, are also forms of speech, and in aphasia (caused by damage to the speech centre in the cerebral cortex) suffer equally with articulate expression and its comprehension. Shelley wrote:

> He gave men speech, and speech created thought,
> Which is the measure of the universe.[8]

It might be argued that we can think in picture images, and often do. Animals think. Yet it is hard to imagine how conceptual thinking can be maintained without the language of concepts, for which no picture image exists. And we need to recall that it is propositions or a series of words in which something is stated, affirmed or denied, not words themselves, that enable the communication of ideas.[9] Even the word 'yes' is a response to something. It is sentences that we recognise, too, rather than individual words. Consider the following:

> Yuo cna raed this wouthit a porbelm.Tihs is bcusease the huamn mnid deos not raed ervey lteter by istlef but the wrod as a wlohe. Amazanig, huh?

Under the British Nationality Act of 1961, an applicant must speak one of three languages native to Great Britain – English, Welsh or Scots Gaelic. Yet there are now over 100 languages in daily use in the UK. Notable among these are both Asian and other European languages – Punjabi, Bengali, Urdu, Gujarati, German, Italian, Polish, Greek, Spanish, Cantonese. Around 25 minority languages are taught in schools to over half a million pupils. Increasing international mobility is likely to make this situation more complex. Personal linguistic identity is closely bound up with ethnic identity (defined as an allegiance to a group with which one has ancestral links), and in its turn with nationhood. Within a language such as English, 'class indicators' identify social identity (upper-class usage differs from others: 'U versus non-U'), and both accent (pronunciation) and dialect (grammar and vocabulary) identify geographical identity. Male and female speech differs, too, although some of this is almost certainly socially determined. Exclamations, emotive adjectives and intensifiers (*so* lovely) differ between men and women.

LANGUAGE AND PERFORMANCE

In a speech made in 1858 for the Royal Theatrical Fund, Charles Dickens remarked that 'Every writer of fiction, though he may not adopt the dramatic form, writes in effect for the stage.' Earlier, William Wordsworth had written:

> My purpose was to imitate and as far as is possible to adopt the very language of men. . . . There will be found in these volumes little of what is usually called poetic diction, as much pains has been taken to avoid it as is ordinarily taken to produce it. . . . It may be safely affirmed that there neither is, nor can be, any essential difference between the language of prose and metrical composition.[10]

For Dickens, language is a performance, and for Wordsworth, prose and poetry are essentially the same.

I have already noted that language has tacit roots. In ordinary discourse, language works in two parts – sense-reading and sense-giving.[11] Sense-reading has to do with the process of discerning the meaning of someone else's utterance, while sense-giving pertains to how it is that a speaker forms a meaningful utterance. In both cases, let us realise that the grasping and imparting of meaning through language is not fundamentally an intellectual process. What is significant in this process is tacit. We tacitly integrate the particulars of our subsidiary awareness by means of our bodily interaction with, or indwelling of them.[12] This is how language works. Gill continues in his exposition:

> Language does not simply float by and through our consciousness as a self-contained entity. On the contrary, it is encountered at the vortex of our involvement with other persons amidst our common tasks in the world around us . . . we get things done with language.[13]

Language is a performance. Just as we integrate the visual clues for perceiving an object, or integrate our muscular contractions when riding a bicycle, while relying on our subsidiary awareness of some things for the purpose of attending focally to a matter on which they bear, so too language is a performance.

NAMING

Naming has been said to be the function of poets and priests. In naming, a word is given to some thing, some thought, some experience or some action. By naming, the experiential is forced into the linguistic. The importance of naming has been recognised for thousands of years. In the Hebrew scriptures, for example, the first task of Adam after the prohibition on eating from the tree of knowledge is to name things:

> He brought them to the man to see what he would call them, and whatever the man called each living creature, that was its name. Thus the man gave names to all cattle, to the birds of heaven, and to every wild animal.[14]

In giving him that power, God gives Adam the possibility of wisdom. Calling things by their right name is the beginning of wisdom for most of us. That link, too, has been recognised by the sages of the civilisations of the Near East. A word spoken at the wrong time threatened the harmony of nature, while in the wisdom literature it was the divine word that created all things.[15] In Christian belief, Christ is seen as the divine creating word – what God was, the Word was.[16] Naming still brings things into existence. As we sicken, we name the sickness and it achieves credibility.

Let us go back to our stories. First we shall consider Liz:

To get out, to be free. . . . To forget that label. Epileptic.

Then Jake:

The skin. The psoriasis. Jake couldn't believe his ears.

Liz has put a name to it. In the narrative, the word occupies a single paragraph of its own. It represents the culmination of that early stage in many experiences of illness. It has this name – this is what it is. In naming it, we begin to understand and, for many, we can interpret in the way that we choose (yes, truly, choose) or have thrust upon us. We bring our own beliefs to that word.

In that naming process, we classify and, in the names we give, we interpret. We describe our symptoms as being due to stress, not due to anxiety. Why? Because stress is what overtakes us as energetic, dedicated, hard-working, integrated people, struggling with the titanic external forces that have finally overcome us. But anxiety? Not the external world that forces our response, but the result of inner weakness, a further collapse of a personality that does not have the strength to cope with the ordinary, the everyday, the banal. Anxiety is a moral judgement on us and a negative one. Stress is, almost, a term of approbation. We were tough enough to face up to *that*. Stress externalises, anxiety internalises. *The gut let him down*, we read in Jake's story. The symptom is distanced – it is a failure of one of my tools, not of me.

Empirical data shed some light on this. One of the many controversies surrounding chronic fatigue syndrome is the possible impact of the diagnostic label. In a narrative synthesis of the literature, it was found that diagnosed patients with a label of chronic fatigue syndrome have a worse prognosis than such patients without a label. The ways in which patients perceive themselves, label their symptoms and appraise stressors may perpetuate or exacerbate their symptoms. This is a process that involves psychological, psychosocial and cultural factors. Finding a label that fits one's condition can provide meaning, emotional relief and recognition, whilst denial can be counter-productive. The answer to the question of whether 'to label or not to label' may turn out to depend not on the label, but on what the label implies.[17]

These issues are most acute in those syndromes that fail to fall into commonly accepted diagnostic categories. Patients with symptoms that are unexplained by disease are particularly likely to be affected by the naming process. Many will have their own views on how that illness should be named. Certain labels carry strongly negative connotations for many patients, implying in their minds that symptoms are imagined or 'put on' or that they are 'mad.' Thus the label 'functional' was found to cause offence to patients far less widely than was the expression 'medically unexplained symptoms', despite the neutral tone of the last phrase.[18] Presumably, 'functional' is at least a positive answer, while 'medically unexplained symptoms' still leaves the suspicion that the explanation is an unacceptable psychological one.

'Hysteria' is a term that specifically excludes malingering, yet it is entirely unacceptable to most patients.[19] In another study it was suggested that media and political pressure can lead to a collusion between patients and doctors. The naming of possibilities gives structure to perceptions and forms the description for behaviour that leads to 'fibromyalgia'.[20] The patient, having gone through this process in the early stage of illness, then has to constantly grow into conformity with classification criteria. The naming process creates the disease, with all of its ramifications.

METAPHOR

As we grow, our vocabulary extends, our experience widens and we become aware of broader and deeper significances in our speech. We grasp the intended meanings of the speaking community in which we find ourselves, and we integrate them, at the tacit level, into significant wholes. Metaphor provides us with excellent examples of this. If we rely on our awareness of something (let us call it A) for attending to something else (let us call it B), we are but subsidiarily aware of A. It is B which is the meaning of A. Although B is always identifiable, A may not always be. In order to grasp the significance of a symbolic expression, we must attend to its meaning through more than the literal meanings of the words involved. 'The pain was a tiger clawing out my chest' tells the doctor the meaning of an intense pain. It does not project the attention of the listener to an enraged wild animal seizing its prey in a clearing in the jungle or a cage in the zoo. Rather, it summarises the intensity of an experience – what it really meant for the sufferer.

Metaphor consists in giving the thing a name that belongs to something else, wrote Aristotle. It is saying one thing, but meaning another. Polanyi and Prosch ask why it is that this 'misnaming' moves us so greatly, and return to Aristotle's assertion that 'a good metaphor implies an intuitive grasp of dissimilars.'[21] Perhaps there is a delight or pleasure in grasping these meanings, rather as there is pleasure in solving a crossword puzzle, speaking another language or talking in cockney rhyming slang. But there is more than this. The good metaphor forces the listener to connect two ideas, the 'from–to' relationship – from the clawing tiger to the meaning that it projects and upon which we focus. It is a tacit process which leads to a meaning that goes beyond the ordinary words of its subsidiary vocabulary. The tiger's claw is an absurd statement if we concentrate on it literally. How could *anyone* know what it would feel like, let alone a retired miner sitting in the Accident and Emergency Department at midnight? It seems implausible that the experience could be survived, and even less likely that it could be solemnly described to assist in the individual's medical history. Yet that is the kind of thing that is said, frequently, colourfully and imaginatively.

Pain – that word that holds a compendium of meanings – more than any other complaint that patients have is often expressed in metaphor or its relative, simile. 'It was like a hammer hitting the back of my head', 'It was a ton weight on my chest', 'It was a tight band so I couldn't breathe', 'It was a toothache in my shoulder', 'It was a sort of boring sensation deep inside.' Note this last example, for the metaphor has almost slipped past the listener unnoticed, as it so often does. Thus we have a series of metaphors that are used to describe health and disease, so familiar – and so subsidiary – that we rarely consider them. There is the military metaphor:

> She is *fighting* for her life.
> The *war* against cancer.
> The *struggle* to pull through.
> The *battle* against the tumour.
> We must *kill* the pain.

Or the mind as a brittle object:[22]

> He had a nervous *breakdown*.
> Since the diagnosis, he's *gone to pieces*.
> I feel pretty *fragile*.
> Doctor, I'm tired, absolutely *shattered*.

What do patients achieve by this? The answer surely is a meaning that could not be achieved without it. 'We have all been prisoners of language too long', wrote RS Thomas. Our vocabulary is insufficient to express those things that are most important to us. Words must therefore be used in ways that make little literal sense – we can imagine a shattered pot, but not a shattered human body. Listening to the patient, the doctor doesn't even think about it.

MEANING, EXPRESSION AND INTENTION

Words change their meaning, too. Words may never be capable of translation from one language to another (for example, the German *gemütlich*, the Welsh *hywl*). Words may have local meanings and usages that are unfamiliar to the health professional arriving from outside a community. 'On times' in Wales has nothing to do with punctuality – rather it means 'occasionally'. Understanding the patient at anything beyond a superficial level may demand a profound cultural understanding.

Our ordinary language gives us clues to the way we use those words with which we present our symptoms. Thus we may say that we 'get it', 'grasp it' or 'see it', as if understanding consisted in possessing or experiencing a mental event or object. Words are noises or marks. The meaning of them is not something that we experience, but something we know from repeated and consistent performance. Consider three kinds of knowing:

1 knowing that something is the case
2 being able to do something (knowing how to do it)
3 knowing some person, place or thing.

Understanding and knowing the meaning of a word is the second sort of knowing. A word is a tool with a certain use, and knowing its meaning is having the skill to use it. Knowing the meaning of a word, like knowing how to swim, is a skill. Literary critics may debate whether the meaning of a word is determined by the writer's intentions, the readers' interpretations, or just the words. 'Daffodil' may communicate a specific meaning to a Wordsworthian, a whip to the kinky, or a worm-eaten carrot to the gardener. Words chosen have different effects on different listeners. Assertions about the associations of words are empirical – sorrow with a nightingale, scarlet with sin, a red rose with love. Narratives of early illness may often be given in a fairly vestigial form, with description of symptoms being fragmentary. Perhaps Rachel will later tell her doctor that she was seized by raging thirst and couldn't go to her violin lesson, and then passed out in the toilet. However, as Greenhalgh and Hurwitz point out, such narratives are a mirror held up to nature. They are closely aligned to physiological and pathological mechanisms, so that the story then linguistically portrays particular biological dysfunctions faithfully.[23]

Here is an illustrative (and true) story. 'The patient is complaining of tinnitus,' reported the young doctor to his senior. 'What do you mean?' inquired the consultant, 'Surely the patient did not say "tinnitus"?' 'No,' came the reply, 'she said that she had ringing in the ears.' The consultant turned to the patient. 'Tell me what you are complaining of.' 'I have ringing in the ears,' she replied. 'Tell me more about it,' he said. 'Well, . . . it's bells . . . church bells . . . playing "Rock of Ages"' [a popular eighteenth-century English hymn].

The direction of inquiry changed, of course – away from the otological to the psychiatric or neurological. The young doctor had failed to understand the metaphor, or rather the lack of it. 'Ringing in the ears' simply meant 'tinnitus'.

In a world of simple expressions, where putting the patient's complaint into a box was more important than exploring it, there was no understanding of metaphor, only a mechanical translation of supposed synonyms.

Disease reduces the capacity for expression. Weariness, exhaustion and malaise reduce the ability to command the range of words formerly at our disposal. Our vocabulary decreases as the process of thinking seemingly requires more work. Damage to the speech centres of the brain is the extreme example of this. Localisation of the functions of speech has been the subject of much controversy. On the one hand, there has been the representation of its different elements in discrete anatomical areas of the brain. On the other, it has been argued that the formulation of propositions in verbal symbols cannot be the function of small isolated portions of the brain. However, it is incontestable that certain areas of damage affect different elements of speech. 'Dysphasia' is the term that refers to the disorder of the symbolic function of speech involved in the comprehension and expression of meaning by means of words. This is usually the result of damage to the left hemisphere of the brain in right-handed people, and in about 60% of left-handed people as well. (Differences occur in the extent of hemisphere dominance for languages, such as Chinese and Japanese, in which there is a pictorial as well as a phonetic component.) Although a general distinction can be made between sensory dysphasia, in which comprehension of the spoken word is lost, and motor dysphasia, in which production of speech is lost, a wide variety of problems are seen in practice, and there is a corresponding debate on the classification of such disorders. Problems may be partial, of course, and the patient who speaks two languages may revert to being able to comprehend or use only the language first learned in childhood, even if they have used the second language for most of their life. Dysphasic patients may use inappropriate words, wrong words, neologisms or more basic noises ('oi, oi, oi' in different tones).Then we have palilalia, dysprosody, semantic paraphasias, the colour and letter anomias, and the concepts of parallel distributed processing across neural networks – the physiological science of speech with its own rich language, whose descriptions can be found neurology texts. Suffice it to observe here that dysphasias may disrupt the expression of meaning even at a level at which the existence of dysphasia is not immediately evident to the unobservant.

Finally, not all matters of health or illness are expressed in words or gestures. Sometimes it is silence that speaks loudest (if the reader will forgive the metaphor). Good communicators understand this. Communication is much more than the transfer of information, and words do not account for all the messages that we communicate. Professionals especially need to reflect on these issues, to acquire the necessary skills,[24] and to reflect on the importance of the vocabulary of disease.

REFERENCES

1 Enright DJ. *The Faber Book of Fevers and Frets*. London: Faber and Faber; 1989.
2 Medawar P, Medawar J. *Aristotle to Zoos. A philosophical dictionary of biology*. Oxford: Oxford University Press; 1985.
3 Kellogg WN, Kellogg LA. *The Ape and the Child*. New York: McGraw-Hill Book Co.; 1933.
4 Polanyi M. *Personal Knowledge: towards a post critical philosophy*. London: Routledge & Kegan Paul; 1958. p. 75.
5 General Medical Council. *Good Medical Practice*. London: General Medical Council; 2001. paragraph 21.
6 Federation of Royal Colleges of Physicians of the UK. *Consultant Physicians Working with Patients*. 3rd ed. London: Royal College of Physicians; 2005.
7 Crystal D. *The Cambridge Encyclopaedia of Language*. 2nd ed. Cambridge: Cambridge University Press; 1997.
8 Shelley PB. Prometheus Unbound. In: *Percy Bysshe Shelley – the Major Works*. Oxford: Oxford University Press; 2003.
9 Holmes G (revised by B Matthews). *Introduction to Clinical Neurology*. 3rd ed. Edinburgh: Churchill Livingstone; 1968.
10 Wordsworth W. Preface to the *Lyrical Ballads*, 1800. In: W Wordsworth, ST Coleridge. *Lyrical Ballads*. London: Penguin Classics; 2007.
11 Polanyi M. Sense-reading and sense-giving. In: Grene M, editor. *Knowing and Being*. London: Routledge & Kegan Paul; 1969. pp. 181–207.
12 Gill JH. *The Tacit Mode*. Albany, NY: State of New York Press; 2000.
13 Gill JH, op. cit.
14 *Genesis 2, 19*; New English Bible translation.
15 *Wisdom of Solomon 9, 1*; New English Bible translation.
16 *John 1, 1*; New English Bible translation.
17 Lakoff G, Johnson M. *Metaphors We Live By*. Chicago: University of Chicago Press; 1980.
18 Stone J, Wojcik W *et al.* What should we say to patients with symptoms unexplained by disease? The 'number needed to offend.' *BMJ*. 2002; **325:** 1449–50.
19 Huibers MJH, Wessely S. The act of diagnosis: pros and cons of labelling chronic fatigue syndrome. *Psychol Med*. Cambridge Journals Online, 10 January 2006.
20 Hazemeijer I, Rasker JJ. Fibromyalgia and the therapeutic domain. A philosophical study on the origins of fibromyalgia in a specific social setting. *Rheumatology*. 2003; **42:** 502–15.
21 Polanyi M, Prosch H. *Meaning*. Chicago: University of Chicago Press; 1975.
22 Stone J, Wojcik W *et al.*, op. cit.
23 Greenhalgh T, Hurwitz B. Why study narrative? *BMJ*. 1999; **318:** 48–50.
24 Simpson M, Buckman R, Stewart M *et al.* Doctor–patient communication: the Toronto consensus statement. *BMJ*. 1991; **303:** 1385–7.

CHAPTER 5

Seeing ourselves: interpreting the visual signs of illness

JANE MACNAUGHTON

INTRODUCTION

'My child's face is disappearing!'

When I picked up the phone late one evening while on call as a general practice trainee, this was all I heard from the distraught mother on the other end of the line. I tried to get her to explain what she was saying in terms that I could understand but she was unable to do so; this was what she was seeing, and she was describing it to me as plainly as she could. I hesitated – it was late, and her house was a long way off – but my hesitation was momentary. This was one of those times when as a clinician you are so struck by the truth of what you are hearing that you know the situation is urgent and probably serious. I went and found a critically dehydrated little girl wandering trance-like between her parents, pale and with deeply sunken features. She turned out to have a blood sugar level ten times what it should have been, and to have developed diabetes.

The clue to this little girl's illness was there in that one sentence of physical description given by her mother. The most important clue, in fact, was in the odd juxtaposition of two apparently unconnected notions: I had not come across the idea that a face might 'disappear.' The language was significant, and I shall return later to discuss the way in which language reveals – in helpful and unhelpful ways – the physical signs of illness.

In this volume we have already discussed the significance for patients of symptoms – the subjective experiences of illness which can vary between sufferers of the same disease. This chapter will deal with visual clues to both health and illness, how we interpret them and what might be the influences upon us as we strive to understand what they mean; and thereafter, what changes in our appearance might require us to seek medical advice. In terms understood by clinicians, such visual clues are regarded as 'signs' (*see* Chapter 7) – something which can be seen, such as a rash, swelling or discoloration. However, patients – or people before they 'become' patients – are the first to discover such signs, to think about them, to discuss them with partners or family, and to come to a conclusion about their significance. The process by which they reach this conclusion is the subject of this chapter.

The 'discovery' of a physical clue to illness may come as a result of a change in appearance, such as the rash of chickenpox or the painless swelling of a tumour in the neck. The rash or swelling thus becomes the pivotal sign that we might now be ill. In some cases the decision that there is a problem and that our body needs treatment may be made only when we realise that there is a treatment available to alleviate the problem. We might think here of cosmetic surgery, which has recently become much more easily accessible and affordable. However, it is the fact of a change that most commonly turns a physical manifestation into a clue that something is wrong. Not all changes, of course, will be seen as signs of possible illness. We accept the kinds of changes that occur, for example, as a result of age, such as wrinkling and spotting of the skin, and loss and greying of the hair. These appearances are acceptable in a person in their sixties or older, but if they were to appear in a child, as in that rare condition, progeria, where the ageing process is speeded up tenfold, the parents would know that there was something wrong. In order to examine what kinds of physical changes we identify as pathological we might first look at what we think of as the appearance of the body in health.

IMAGES OF HEALTH

Jake is a young man who is concerned with his image. The reader is immediately aware that he is attracted to Carol, and the dramatic tension developed by his reluctance to respond to her invitation is not relieved until the porter gives us an explanation for his reticence: 'The skin. The psoriasis.' For Jake, lusting after Carol but acutely embarrassed about the idea of taking his clothes off in front of anyone (access to 'his own shower' is a huge relief to him), the psoriasis *is* 'the end of the world.' His physical appearance is not described to us but it is enough that the porter notices it. The fact that skin problems may be common ('there's a lot of it about') does not help. Jake sees his appearance as not just scaly and red, and therefore unhealthy, but also as sexually unattractive and undesirable.

In this section I wish to explore further some ideas from a number of literary and other sources about how Western society views the body in health. These examples will show how difficult an idea this is to capture. but also that there may be many influences on our notions of what the appearance of health might be.

Vivid pictures of health are not easy to find in literary sources, although writers will often use illness to explore notions of what health means. Images of illness and death are much more common.[1] This is because experiences of disease and illness are intense and have a certain duration. They thus become objects of attention in their own right and generate a rich variety of images. Writing about illness is intrinsically much more interesting than writing about health, because it is about change and response to change. Health, on the other hand, is regarded as the body's status quo. Being healthy might just be a way of saying that we are not ill or diseased. Medical practice seems to support this view of health, in that the treatment that restores us to health is really just removing disease or illness. Even if we insist that there is more to health than the absence of something – that it refers to some biological balance or equilibrium – we still do not have a concept that is likely to stimulate the imagination of a writer. For when we are in this state of bodily equilibrium – when we are healthy – we do not notice our health but concentrate on other matters instead.

The often quoted 1946 World Health Organization definition of health offers another sense of health:

> Health is a state of complete physical, mental and social well-being, and not just the absence of disease and infirmity.[2]

However, this definition does not really get us very far. While claiming to give a positive character to health, it still does not give health a clear identity, any more than the medical 'absence of disease' or new age 'equilibrium' views of health. For what has come to be known as 'positive health' is a concept in perpetual disguise. It is conceptually impossible to distinguish positive health from other states, such as well-being, happiness, exhilaration, fitness or vigour. In other words, if we want to examine what we understand by the appearance of positive health, we must look for this under other descriptions and guises.

Typically, images of health are presented in terms of youth, beauty and vigour, as in the poem 'The Olympic Girl' by John Betjeman (1906–84).

> The sort of girl I like to see
> Smiles down from her great height at me.
> She stands in strong athletic pose
> And wrinkles her *retroussé* nose . . .
>
> . . .
>
> Little, alas, to you I mean.
> For I am bald and old and green.[3]

The 'strong athletic' youthful girl is contrasted with the 'bald and old' poet, but his 'greenness' reflects the poignant fact that his desire for the girl is unlikely to be requited. Betjeman's girl has much in common with the models whose impossibly slim bodies and perfect complexions bombard us from advertising hoards all over our towns and cities. These carefully airbrushed images are powerful sources for our modern view of what a healthy body should look like.[4] But not all images of healthy bodies are dominated by youth. The late artist Beryl Cook specialised in images of people participating in sports and having a good time. However, in her version of a tennis match entitled *Mixed Doubles*, the participants in the game are not young and slim, but grey, balding and overweight. In other pictures her characters' exuberant enjoyment of life seems to be enhanced rather than diminished by their appetites for alcohol, cigarettes and food.[5] To the viewer, these pictures epitomise a 'healthy' enjoyment of the pleasures of living.

Tolstoy's *War and Peace* uses images of youth, vigour and health as metaphors for moral goodness. In Book One we are introduced to the young people of the Rostov family and in particular to the eldest son, Nicolas, who is described as follows:

> . . . short with curly hair and an open expression. Dark hairs were already showing on his upper lip, and his whole face expressed impetuosity and enthusiasm.[6]

Later, when he joins the army to campaign in the war against Napoleon, we are again struck by his appearance:

> Rostov in his cadet uniform, with a jerk to his horse rode up the porch, swung his leg over the saddle with a supple youthful movement, stood for a moment in the stirrup as if loath to part from his horse, and at last sprang down and called to his orderly.

His sister, Natasha, is similarly portrayed as bursting with good humour and impetuous vitality:

> She . . . glanced up at her younger brother, who was screwing up his eyes and, shaking with suppressed laughter, unable to control herself any longer, she jumped up and rushed from the room as fast as her nimble little feet would carry her.

These attractive portraits follow immediately on from the opening scenes of the novel, which take place at an evening party attended by the aristocracy of St Petersburg. These characters are portrayed as older, false and manipulative. The contrast is striking.

From these examples it emerges that what we consider to be the image of a healthy body may not amount to any one idea, but may be influenced by the concept of 'health' that we hold at that time. Our appreciation of the 'Olympic Girl' is aesthetic: we admire her strong limbs and athletic pose. The concept of health involved here is that of health as beauty. However, that sense of beauty can be contested. We can appreciate the beauty of the sensuous curve of voluptuous flesh in a painting, but do we regard such beauty as 'healthy'? In Beryl Cook's images, our concept of what is healthy is related to enjoyment and *joie de vivre* – the bright smiles of the characters in her paintings are related to good conversation and laughter over a drink and a smoke in the pub. The idea of health here is related to living well, having friends and being able to enjoy communal activities. Finally, the concept of health epitomised by images of the young Rostovs, compared with those of degenerate high society in St Petersburg, is dominated by moral values. Vigorous good health and youth are equated with innocence and goodness. Our view of health, therefore, is affected by our values, aesthetic and moral. Thus our tendency to notice or not notice a physical change as signalling potential illness is affected by these as well.

How do these factors help to determine our views on ill health and its physical manifestations? Other factors are also involved in this process. A lump appearing on our body will give cause for alarm regardless of how our view of health or ill health is determined. The sinking of a child's features and pallor of her skin would always be worrying signs. I shall return to this question later but let us now turn to an examination of the values and other influences that may affect our views of health and disease.

WHAT INFLUENCES OUR VIEWS ABOUT PHYSICAL APPEARANCE?

The science of medicine has had a significant effect on our views about the body from the late nineteenth century.[7] Medical technologies such as X-rays and, more recently and vividly, computed tomography (CT) scans have had a profound effect on our ability to visualise our inner bodies. The dominance of medicine has tended to lead to a medicalisation of some ordinary experiences, such as childbirth, and to an expectation that there is an expert solution to all of life's problems. In my discussion of 'images of health' above, I have even suggested that our concept of what it is to live an enjoyable life has been usurped by a medicalised notion of the 'healthy' life. However, that dominance is now being slowly challenged by the rise of consumer culture in most western societies, with its emphasis on patients' rights[8] and on the relationship between doctor and patient as one of partnership rather than paternalism. The pervasiveness of medical values and of a medical world view on our notions of health and illness will, more appropriately, be the subject of a later volume. Here I wish to concentrate first on two kinds of layman's judgement that we use to make decisions about our appearance and that of others – aesthetic and moral judgements. I shall then discuss what kinds of influences might affect how those judgements are made.

Aesthetic judgements

Aesthetic judgements are integral to our decisions as to whether physical appearances are 'right' or 'wrong.' We frequently describe a rash as 'ugly' (and Jake feels that his rash makes him ugly and undesirable), or say that our joints have become 'disfigured' by arthritis. It is important first to be clear about what we mean here by aesthetic judgements. One view, following Hegel,[9] is that aesthetics is concerned only with art. Another view, that of Kant,[10] regarded aesthetic judgement as including nature as well as art. In Kant's view, aesthetics concerns anything that constitutes an aesthetic experience or that gives 'delight' or is appreciated as beautiful. That aesthetic appreciation is defined as being good, delightful or beautiful in itself and not simply by reason of its usefulness.

Kant's wider view that aesthetic judgements concern more than just art is the one I wish to concentrate on here. The history of art may have been influential in setting standards for what we regard as beauty in the human form, and in reflecting society's *mores* in that respect, but our views about our own and others' bodies have more to do with a sense of what does – or does not – delight the eye. Furthermore, aesthetic judgements in Kant's sense are about a subjective response to (usually) visual experiences, but it is expected that this subjective response would be shared by others and not be unique.

Thus there has to be some agreement in the appreciation of what is beautiful or good in the object – or person – under examination.

Greek philosophers also discussed questions of aesthetics, although not under that name. For Aristotle, beauty was intimately concerned with function and 'fit':

> Beauty for a youth is to have a body suited to work where running and where force is required. Such a body is pleasant, and so enjoyable to look at. (This is why pentathletes are the most beautiful people, since they require both speed and strength.) For a man in the prime of life, beauty is to have a body fitted for the toils of warfare. Such a body seems pleasant, but also formidable. For an old man, beauty is to have a body capable of doing what is essential. Such a body is free of pain, having escaped the ravages of old age.[11]

In Kant's view, what is beautiful and 'right' is what is beautiful in and for itself, and not for any purpose. For Aristotle, function is important. The beauty of the youth derives from the fact that he can do what it is that a young man should be able to do – that is, be an athlete – whereas the old man is expected to live a gentler life, and his body should be fit for conversation and light work.

In making judgements about the appearance of our bodies we tend to bring both of these views together. The swollen, red knee joint of acute arthritis is not pleasant to look at, and it does not function as it should in that it cannot bear our weight. We also have a sense of what is appropriate for our bodies to look like at various stages of life. Returning to the example of Natasha Rostov, Tolstoy describes her appearance after her second marriage as follows:

> She had grown stouter and broader, so that it was hard to recognise in the robust-looking young mother the slim, mobile Natasha of old days. Her features had become more defined, and wore an expression of calm softness and serenity. Her face had no longer that ever-glowing fire of eagerness that had once constituted her chief charm. Now, often her face and body were all that was to be seen, and the soul was not visible at all. All there was to be seen in her was a vigorous, handsome and fruitful mother.[12]

Natasha remains beautiful in later life, but that beauty derives from her role now as a young wife and mother and is appropriate to it. Tolstoy is rather wistful about this, but it is nevertheless clear that the fiery impetuousness of the youthful Natasha would be unfitting in the grown woman.

In summary, our views about how bodies should look and move are partly determined by aesthetic judgements, and these are affected by what we think is appropriate to particular ages and stages in life. The mother who described her daughter's face as 'disappearing' obviously noticed a change, but had also had an aesthetic template in her mind in which healthy 6-year-olds had plump cheeks and ruddy complexions and the little girl's pallor and sunken features departed from that ideal. We all hold these templates in our minds, but those 'healthy' or desirable templates can be affected by influences from the societies in which we live. In 1997, a notorious set of pictures employed to advertise Calvin Klein clothes featured pale, skinny models with dark sunken eyes who looked as if they were drug addicts. The picture led to a craze in the USA for what was dubbed 'heroin chic'. The craze was short-lived, but it illustrated that what we regard as beautiful or fitting or even healthy may be affected by cultural trends and norms. Twenty-first-century Western society suffers from the problems of affluence, including overeating and obesity. Thinness is regarded not as failure but as an achievement, and this is part of the attraction of these controversial images. I shall return to this point in more detail later.

Moral judgements

It is difficult to avoid using the terms 'right' and 'wrong' when describing someone's appearance, as in 'He just did not look right' or 'He was so pale there must have been something wrong'. These senses of 'right' and 'wrong' have more to do with the aesthetic judgements that I have just discussed than any moral judgement about the person concerned. However, moral judgements are often invoked when we consider appearance. Aristotle was clear that physical appearance reflected moral status:

> A small face is a sign of a petty soul . . . a large face means lethargy. . . . So the face must be neither large nor small: an intermediate size is therefore best. (811b 9–11)

> Too much hair on breast and belly mean lack of persistence . . . but breasts too devoid of hair indicate impudence (as in women). So both extremes are bad, and an intermediate condition must best. (812b 14–19)[13]

This idea was further developed in eighteenth-century Europe in the so-called science of phrenology, which mapped the physical appearance and contours of the skull (reflecting the underlying structure of the brain) to the person's personality or moral status.[14] In this case, moral judgements were part of a process of deciding whether an individual was sick and needed treatment or not. The treatments involved here included cold showers and isolation in order to develop moral character.

Such ideas and treatment approaches in psychiatry have long been discredited but moral judgements still feature in our views about whether a body is healthy or not. However, when it comes to our views about whether our appearance or that of others constitutes ill health, moral judgements stand in a different relation from aesthetic judgements. Consider the example of obesity. When we observe someone who is fat (particularly if we ourselves are not), we regard that person as someone who has failed morally in that they have been greedy. We may consider that their obesity may put their health in danger but that view is not integral to our judgement that they are obese. An aesthetic judgment (from a Western perspective) would be that fat is ugly and inappropriate to good human functioning and therefore it needs treatment. The aesthetic value is here integral to the sense that something is amiss with that person.

Rather than assisting a person in seeking treatment, the fact that certain physical states are judged by society as 'morally bad' will often discourage patients from doing anything about them. Obesity is one example where the viewer may feel that it is the obese person's 'fault' and therefore up to them to do something about it. This is despite the fact that the NHS in the UK now runs obesity clinics where such people can receive expensive treatments, such as stomach stapling, free of charge.

There is a strong historical relationship between skin lesions and sexual behaviour that is regarded as morally corrupt. One patient of mine, a middle-aged British man who had just returned from working in southern Africa, delayed seeking treatment for advanced AIDS because of the moral censure on that disease and only presented when his face was distorted by numerous cranial nerve palsies and he was barely able to walk.

Jake's embarrassment about his skin condition may be partly due to echoes of this relationship. Secondary syphilis manifests itself by a rash consisting of red scaly bumps (the pox[15]), and congenital syphilis has characteristic facial features. AIDS also has skin manifestations such as the skin cancer, Kaposi's sarcoma. It has been suggested, particularly by those who hold fundamentalist Christian beliefs, that AIDS is 'God's judgement on homosexual men.' This view has parallels with views about, and approaches to, the public health management of syphilis in the past.[16]

As was the case with aesthetic judgements, moral judgements are affected by concurrent societal and cultural views.

Social and cultural influences on our view of the body

Cecil Helman, general practitioner and anthropologist, emphasises the importance of the influence of our societies and culture on our views of our bodies, stating that:

> . . . each human being has, in a sense, two bodies: an *individual* body-self (both physical and psychological) which is acquired at birth, and also the *social* body that it needs in order to live within a particular society.[17]

At the beginning of this chapter, I discussed how a change in the body's appearance might lead the individual to realise that there was something amiss. However, for most of this chapter I have been dealing with the notion of the social body and how that body is constructed for the individual from external influences. Helman makes reference to the ways in which aesthetic values may differ between societies, and how these may impact on what might be regarded as 'normal' bodily appearances. In Imperial China the feet of little girls were tightly bound to restrict their growth because that society values dainty feet in their women. And the practice in some tribes in Brazil, East Africa and Melanesia of inserting large ornaments into the lips and earlobes reflects an aesthetic preference for enlarged lips and earlobes.[18]

These changes to the body are all effected artificially but some natural bodily states can be regarded as 'abnormal' or even 'unhealthy' as a result of cultural values. Again, obesity is a good example. In some parts of West Africa rich families send their daughters to 'fattening houses' to be fed on excess food and allowed minimal exercise[19] because in that society plump women are valued as reflecting the family's wealth and the individual woman's childbearing capacity, both good ways of attracting a well-to-do mate. This attitude contrasts starkly with the view of Western societies, which value slimness to such an extent that at least 30% of women and 16% of men report trying to diet within a 10-year period.[20] Clearly, different standards of beauty and aesthetic values are involved here, but also different ideas of what constitutes a healthy body. The African view that plumpness reflects healthy fertility is contrasted with the Western view that obesity is a major health problem.

These distinctions reflect widely differing cultural contexts, but it is also possible to detect alterations within Western societies with regard to our notions of what is a healthy body. As people are now beginning to live longer our ideas of what is appropriate for a 60-year-old or even 70-year-old body are changing. We expect people of that age to be more active, slim and youthful in appearance, now that life expectancy for women in the UK is (on average) 81 years and that for men is 75 years.[21] The increasing availability and acceptability of cosmetic surgery is another cultural change that is supporting this alteration in expectations.

Shifts in assumptions about physical appearance have also come about through concerted efforts by pressure groups. One example of this is the disability lobby. Over the last two decades there has been a major shift in our conceptualisation of disability from a medical problem, in which disability is perceived as a somatic and intellectual abnormality,[22] to seeing it as a normal state which the environment should accommodate to allow disabled people to function within it. The language now used to describe disabled people reflects this shift in view – from 'mentally defective', 'moron' and 'cripple' to 'learning disabled', 'disabled' and even 'less abled', now the preferred sign on public toilets for the disabled.

In this section I have focused on what might influence our view of our bodies. These influences can come from the kinds of values that we hold, both aesthetic and moral, and these relate to the prevailing values of our society: cultural, social and political. Reactions to those 'social bodies' that exist alongside our physical bodies can be powerful agencies in our decisions as to whether we are ill.

HOW OTHERS SEE US

> 'You are looking rather pale: are you sure you are all right?'
>
> 'That mole is getting bigger. Don't you think you should get it seen to?'
>
> 'The skin. The psoriasis. . . . It's not the end of the world.'

The responses of others to our physical appearance can have a powerful effect in confirming that we are in fact ill. Turning up at work with a heavy cold only to be met with the comment 'You look dreadful' can immediately make us feel much worse and send us scurrying home to bed. Societal and family influences may mean that one person's heavy cold (with red-rimmed eyes, dripping nose and flushed complexion) may equate with another person's flu. Our views of ourselves and others' views of us may be very different.

This point is best made with reference to some literary examples. In Virginia Woolf's novel about a day in the life of its eponymous heroine, Mrs Dalloway, we experience the power of Woolf's 'stream of consciousness' style when in the first couple of pages we are given two very different views of Clarissa Dalloway.[23] At first we are privy to her own thoughts as she prepares to step out on a June morning to buy flowers for her evening party, while in the background workmen are removing doors in the house in preparation:

> What a lark! What a plunge! For so it had always seemed to her when, with a little squeak of the hinges, which she could hear now, she had burst open the

French windows and plunged at Bourton into the open air.

Then, as she proceeds on her way to collect the flowers:

> She stiffened a little on the kerb, waiting for Durtnall's van to pass. A charming
> woman, Scrope Purves thought her (knowing her as one does know people
> who live next door to one in Westminster); a touch of the bird about her, of
> the jay, blue-green, light, vivacious, though she was over fifty, and grown very
> white since her illness. There she perched, never seeing him, waiting to cross,
> very upright.

Our first idea of Clarissa Dalloway is gained from the perspective of her memory
of herself as a young girl of eighteen; vigorous, 'plunging' out into the morning
air at the country house at which she stayed in the summer, full of life but at
the same time 'solemn', expecting 'something awful to happen', in some ways
also tentative and scared of life. From this we zoom forward to the present day
when abruptly the perspective of the narration is taken over by her neighbour.
The tentativeness seems to have taken over and the vision we now have of
Clarissa is of a vivacious but birdlike woman, slight and ill and ageing.

Another account that contrasts the internal view of oneself with that of outsiders is in a short story by Helen Simpson, *Getting a Life*.[24] We meet Dorrie, the
young mother of the story, glorying in a brief moment of solitary pleasure:

> Dorrie stood at the edge of the early morning garden and inhaled a column
> of chilly air. After the mulch of soft sheets and stumbling down through the
> domestic rubble and crumbs and sleeping bodies, it made her gasp with
> delight . . .

Just after glimpsing Dorrie as someone with an attractive soul, capable of
experiencing joy in a glimpse of the early morning, we have this perspective
from others:

> Nowadays those few who continued to see Dorrie at all registered her as a
> gloomy timid woman who had grown rather fat and overprotective of her
> three infants. . . . She was never still, she was always available, a conciliatory
> twittering fusspot.

As the story progresses, we gather that this view is also shared by her husband
Max, who is unable to glimpse the woman who can glory in a breath of morning air.

What these examples show is that what can be seen of a person from the outside may not necessarily reflect how that person views him- or herself. This is particularly true of psychological states but may also be so of physical states. It is not uncommon for elderly people to complain that they find it difficult to recognise the old face they see in the mirror: 'I still feel the way I did in my twenties!' Clarissa Dalloway may appear sick and 'birdlike', but inside she is still retains part of that 18-year-old starting out in life with tentative hope. Our views of ourselves clothe our bodies with a number of identities which are not recognisable to outsiders but which may be important to understand if – as doctors – we wish to help those whose illnesses have a significant effect on their physical appearance. This idea is represented in the following poem, 'Ways of Discussing My Body', by Julia Darling,[25] who herself died of breast cancer in her late forties:

> I am a cow, when her calves are taken,
> mooing by the gate, with muddy knees.
> I'm a woodshed before the explosion,
> a swollen kite, pulling at a string.
> A giraffe with a narrow and fragile neck,
> a still life that's shabbily arranged,
> a badly made stool that won't stand up.
> I'm that pair of uncomfortable shoes.
> I'm a soldier, a veil. I'm a wardrobe.
> Do you understand me? I am not what you see.
> I am buried at the bottom of a lake.
> My parts are many and they don't match.

The poet urgently requests that her family, friends and medical attendants attempt to understand her physical state. However, that state and the psychological disintegration that goes with it are so complex and ever-changing that such understanding seems impossible. She asks them to understand that what they see is not her – or even the summation of her illness – but a complex mix of symptoms, signs and feelings that do not add up or make sense.

Modern medical technology has become increasingly concerned with describing the human body in a code created by combining the letters C, A G and T: the first letters of the proteins that make up the molecules of the genetic code. The body here described is an abstraction – a statistical or diagrammatic averaging of the body rather than a reflection of the true complexity of living, breathing, interacting flesh in the world. The vocabulary of science is not sufficient to describe and capture its complexity. Our nearest and dearest family and friends are often more accurate in their attempts to capture the truth of what our external appearance is signalling about our bodies. 'My daughter's face is disappearing' is an eerily accurate description. Literature reminds us that what can be described about our external appearance from the outside by others needs to be checked against our own views and feelings.

SUMMARY

This chapter has explored some of the influences on the ways in which we perceive our physical status. If our bodies become ill, our first perception may be of a change in appearance, but in order to perceive this we must have some idea of what a 'normal' healthy body looks like. The appearance of health and ill health may vary depending on our own aesthetic and moral values and on the cultural norms and assumptions of the society in which we live. Those influences feed into the views that others may have of our 'illness appearance', which may be at odds with our experiences as a patient. They may also affect how we feel and what we go on to do about it. In the next chapter we shall explore in more detail the response of others to illness, disease and suffering.

REFERENCES

1 Downie RS, Macnaughton J. Images of health. *Lancet.* 1998; **351:** 823–5.
2 World Health Organization. *Constitution.* New York: World Health Organization; 1946.
3 Betjeman J. The Olympic Girl. In: *Collected Poems.* London: John Murray; 1958.
4 Jagger E. Consumer bodies. In: Hancock P *et al.,* editors. *The Body, Culture and Society: an introduction.* Buckingham: Open University Press; 2000. pp. 45–63.
5 Cook B. *Happy Days.* London: Victor Gollancz; 1995.
6 Tolstoy L (Maude L, Maude A, trans.). *War and Peace.* Oxford: Oxford University Press; 1922.
7 Hancock P *et al.,* editors. *The Body, Culture and Society: an introduction.* Buckingham: Open University Press; 2000. p. 6.
8 Department of Health. *The Patient's Charter.* London: Department of Health; 1991.
9 Hegel GWF. *Introduction to Aesthetics* (Trans. TM Knox). Oxford: Clarendon Press; 1975, pp. 1–14.
10 Kant I. *Critique of Judgement.* (Trans. JC Meredith). Oxford: Clarendon Press; 1952, Sections 1–14.
11 Aristotle. *Rhetoric,* 1.5, 1361b 7–14. (Quoted by G Boys Stones. 'Polyclitus among the philosophers: canons of classical beauty'. In: C Saunders, U Maude, J Macnaughton (eds) *The Body and the Arts.* London: Palgrave; 2008.)
12 Tolstoy L, op. cit., p. 1247.
13 Aristotle. *Physiognomy.* (Quoted by G Boys Stones. 'Polyclitus among the philosophers:

canons of classical beauty'. In: C Saunders, U Maude, J Macnaughton (eds) *The Body and the Arts*. London: Palgrave; 2008.)

14 Porter R. *The Greatest Benefit to Mankind*. London: HarperCollins; 1997. pp. 499–500.

15 Ibid., pp. 421, 451.

16 Treadwell P. *God's Judgement. Syphilis and AIDS*. Lincoln: Writers Club Press; 2001.

17 Helman CG. *Culture, Health and Illness*. 2nd ed. London: Wright; 1990. p. 14.

18 Helman CG, op. cit., p. 13.

19 Helman CG, op. cit., p. 13.

20 Provencher V *et al*. Eating behaviours, dietary profile and body composition according to dieting history in men and women of the Quebec Family Study. *Br J Nutr*. 2004; **91**: 997–1004.

21 National Statistics Online.

22 Paterson K, Hughes B. Disabled bodies. In: Hancock P *et al*., editors. *The Body, Culture and Society: an introduction*. Buckingham: Open University Press; 2000. pp. 29–44.

23 Woolf V. *Mrs Dalloway*. London: Granada Publishing Ltd; 1976. p. 5.

24 Simpson H. *Getting a Life*. New York: Vintage Books; 2000. pp. 27–64.

25 Darling J. *Apology for Absence*. Todmorden: Arc Publishing; 2004.

CHAPTER 6

The response to suffering

JILL GORDON

In *A Prayer for my Son*,[1] WB Yeats expresses an anxious concern that is immediately recognisable to the parents of the very young:

> Bid a strong ghost stand at the head
> That my Michael may sleep sound
> Nor cry, nor turn in the bed
> Till his morning meal come round.

The supernatural strength and protection afforded by a 'strong ghost' must have been the devout wish of any parent who, in 1928, when this poem was published, knew that early death was commonplace. In England and Wales, seven or eight infant boys died for every hundred boys born, a significantly higher rate than mortality in infant girls.[2] The figures could only have been worse for Ireland. Perhaps this is why Yeats, while still conveying his anxiety and protectiveness in *A Prayer for My Daughter*, nevertheless envisages her life right through to the moment when her bridegroom will take her safely to *'a house/where all's accustomed, ceremonious.'*

How does an inexperienced father know whether baby Michael has a serious illness?

> You have lacked articulate speech
> To tell Your simplest want.

Here is a poignant example of the emotional upheaval that can be caused by observing and trying to interpret the experience of another. Even between adults with full powers of expression, the incommensurability of human experience and the incommunicability of suffering make it difficult to find the 'right' response to another in distress.

Rachel, Jake, Liz and Jen are all involved in relationships. The symptoms that they experience are affecting not only themselves, but also the people who are important in their lives, even before the symptoms are fully recognised, revealed and discussed. Each of the characters in our stories has already altered their behaviour as a result of their symptoms, and this in turn has had an effect on their relationships with others. Rachel's tiredness evokes her mother's incredulous response 'You want to go to bed?' Her brother Alex is frustrated by the unexplained disappearance of some Coke reserved for a party, and by the fact that Rachel keeps commandeering the bathroom where he wants to preen in preparation for meeting his girlfriend. Jake is embarrassed by his gut symptoms, and his behaviour makes his girlfriend wonder whether or not he is really interested in her. Liz's status as a single mother, whose ex-husband has questioned her ability to cope alone with their daughter Sophie, causes her to try to ignore the headache and the aura that warn of the possibility of an epileptic seizure. Jen can barely find the energy to respond to her husband Geoff's demands. Each of them is teetering on the edge between wellness, or relative wellness, and sickness. Each of them is changing in ways that affect other people. This chapter considers symptoms in terms of their effects on relationships – the response to suffering. It looks in particular at the factors that bear on the relationship between the sufferer and significant others.

THE DECISION TO TELL

The preceding chapters have dealt with an inner experience that involves decision making, and this inner experience and decision-making process often develop in the form of a dialogue. We talk to ourselves as much as, or more than, we talk to those around us. Because it is difficult to be objective about one's own symptoms, the doctor who treats his own condition is said to have a fool for a physician. This loss of objectivity applies to lay people as well as doctors. The way out of this 'foolishness' is to enlist the help of others in interpreting our symptoms, and to use them as reference points for a more rational approach to illness.

Each individual responds to symptoms according to his or her personality and life experiences. The individual who is prone to 'catastrophising' may bring to mind the worst-case scenario, whereas a more phlegmatic individual may be inclined to minimise the significance of any symptoms. Once the viewpoints of others are introduced, these personal characteristics tend to be diluted, and this may help or impair the process of deciding what to do next. Other people's responses to our symptoms can have a critically important effect on outcomes. Doctors not infrequently encounter patients who did not intend to do anything about a potentially serious symptom, until a worried family member insisted that they saw a doctor.

Rachel is only 10 years old, and feels confused by the recent change in her appetite and thirst and by her increasing fatigue. She is in particular danger because she is unlikely to realise that the symptoms are serious and that she should tell her mother what is happening to her. Why she hides her symptoms is unclear, but her own personality and perhaps her mother's distractedness are clues. Rachel may not want to be the cause of more worry for her busy mum.

Jake feels ashamed of having a disfiguring condition like psoriasis and an embarrassing one like irritable bowel syndrome. Liz feels vulnerable as a single mother with epilepsy, a situation that probably exacerbates her already negative attitude towards a routine cervical cancer smear. Jen has adapted to the life of the martyr, and may dread having to talk to Geoff about her own needs.

At this stage, each of them is facing a risk. Will their concerns elicit sympathy or blame? Will they be trivialised? Will the other person remind them that they have neglected themselves in some way and that they 'deserve' the symptoms?

All of these risks are further complicated when significant psychological, social, cultural or religious differences are involved. Some cultural groups have firm beliefs about sharing concerns within families, especially when it comes to telling a family member that they have a serious disease.[3] In cultures that are highly communitarian, the diagnosis may be kept hidden from the sufferer, while more individualistic cultures may tend to encourage disclosure and place the burden of responsibility for dealing with illness more firmly on the shoulders of the sufferer.

It is possible to identify quite different perspectives on that moment prior to the disclosure of a health concern. What might be happening from an existential, evolutionary, sociological, psychological or relational perspective?

THROUGH AN EXISTENTIAL LENS

In the context of our discussion of symptoms, existential psychiatry can provide a way of appreciating what happens when individuals share the struggle to make sense of their worlds. Existential psychiatry emerged from the work of Erich Fromm,[4] Jean-Paul Sartre[5] and others. In clinical psychiatry it has been revived by psychiatrists such as Irvin Yalom,[6] who set it against Freudian approaches and the anti-intellectual forms of humanistic therapy, both of which have failed to demonstrate significant advantages over what has been termed simply 'good clinical care.'[7] It is a clinical approach that recognises as major causes of anxiety the questions posed by our mortality, freedom of choice, isolation and life meaning. These concerns can be considered not only from the perspective of the individuals who are experiencing symptoms, but also from the perspective of those who are involved in relationships with them.

Mortality

A new symptom carries with it the possibility of a serious illness and even death. The fear of death is ever present for adult humans, and is present for children from quite a young age. We come to terms with the reality of death over an entire lifetime, succeeding in ignoring it for much of our lives, but occasionally caught out perhaps when a loved one or a person with whom we share certain characteristics dies. The death of a colleague or a contemporary is often a powerful reminder of our own mortality.

A symptom can awaken a sense of vulnerability, and as soon as it is communicated to others, it becomes a reminder of their vulnerability as well.

Rachel is not aware that her symptoms and their implications could be very serious, but her parents certainly will be, and inevitably they will communicate their anxiety to her. It will be extremely difficult for them not to over-react to the diagnosis, with its implications for insulin therapy, hypo- and hyperglycaemic reactions, and the possibility of long-term complications. This is perhaps the most dramatic example among the four stories – all the more so because Rachel is a child and her diagnosis is potentially so serious.

Jake, on the other hand, is not going to die unless we count 'dying' of embarrassment. We get the feeling from this story that Carol's common-sense approach will be instrumental in releasing Jake from some of his embarrassment and enabling him to develop more self-confidence, based on the fact that at least one woman in the world fancies him!

Liz could indeed die as a result of epilepsy, but this is unlikely. Far worse for her is the thought of her own helplessness and lack of autonomy when 'taken' by a seizure. To a large extent, we suspect that she is more worried about her daughter's safety and well-being than her own. To experience epilepsy is to experience loss of control. What if she had an extended period in which her seizures were hard to manage? Could her ex-husband argue a case for taking Sophie away from her? Here an intimate relationship that turned sour defines a large measure of Liz's response to her symptoms.

Jen knows very well that her symptom may be connected to a very serious illness, and that sharing this information with her disabled husband will have profound ramifications. It may well prove to be the single biggest test of their relationship. Will he respond with the question 'What will happen to me now?' or will it be 'What can I do to help you?' or simply 'We'll face this together'.

Personal freedom

The second major existential issue is personal freedom. Erich Fromm wrote about 'the fear of freedom'[4] because he recognised the lengths to which humans will go to achieve certainty, even if the certainty requires them to relinquish their freedom. Freedom to chart our own course reminds us that we could choose the 'wrong' path (i.e. a path that takes us closer to death). A symptom requires us to choose a course of action or inaction. Will it be the 'right' choice? How will significant others respond to the choices that we make? How will they contribute to the decision-making process? Will they try to curtail our freedom?

As a child, Rachel is the least free, but if a diagnosis of diabetes is confirmed, her parents may still be faced with the problem of ensuring that she complies with treatment. If Rachel is resistant or forgetful, how far should they go to force her to use her insulin at the right time, to exercise and eat according to an ideal routine, and to take special care of herself in a number of other ways? Will her teachers and others also join in the task of limiting her freedom?

Jake's freedom includes the freedom to hide his symptoms and put his relationship with Carol at risk. At the moment, Carol seems to be intent on limiting his freedom in a way that Jake himself finds very appealing, but what if she were to go too far and demand more intimacy than Jake is capable of sharing with her? In fact, his 'freedom' to hide his symptoms is really a form of confinement, since our story makes it clear that he would dearly love to have a closer relationship with her.

Liz is well aware that her day-to-day freedom is limited by her responsibility to care for Sophie. She cannot afford to do anything that might lead her to lose her daughter. Now she confronts choices in which Sophie is a key factor – and by ignoring her symptoms, Liz may be risking her custody more than if she moved quickly to clarify what is happening to her.

Jen's freedom is the most severely restricted of the four. She is afraid of the impact of illness not only on herself, but also on Geoff. To complicate matters, her feelings towards Geoff are ambivalent. Paradoxically, her illness may afford her greater freedom than wellness can offer, by releasing her from some of her obligations to deal sympathetically with Geoff and his disabilities.

Personal isolation

No one can fully communicate their experience of being; we are each cut off from the other when it comes to sharing our innermost thoughts and feelings. This existential isolation can be ameliorated or worsened by the impact of illness. In Rachel's case, finding a cause for her odd behaviour is likely to make her feel less isolated. The early symptoms of diabetes may cause confusion for both existential and biochemical reasons. Once an explanation is found, her parents and other family members are likely to pay her special attention, and she may feel less alone. For the patients in the other stories, there are serious risks. There is a possibility that revealing their symptoms may result in greater isolation.

Identifying meaning

As we saw in Chapter 1, of all of the challenges to our illusion of order and purpose in life, the sudden advent of symptoms is probably one of the greatest. The question 'Why me?' has, embedded within it, the assumption that life has meaning and that events occur for a reason. Few people are able to ask the equally valid question 'Why not me?' Symptoms tend to be accompanied by a search for explanations – a something or someone to blame. Long before Job plumbed the depths of suffering, humans tended to link illness to the disapproval of God or the gods, or to apportion blame to the sufferer. For many people, the explanation of suffering needs to encompass both the biomedical and the existential. Revealing one's symptoms to others means opening up to accusations which can carry echoes of ancient superstitions. Even when they are dressed up in modern clothing ('Your lifestyle has contributed to your symptoms'), there is a sense of predestination – the same sense that is invoked by Yeats' anxious musings about his son. The nursery is crowded; as well as father and child, there are 'devilish things' that seek revenge for sins yet to be committed:

> Bid the ghost have sword in fist:
> Some there are, for I avow
> Such devilish things exist,
> Who have planned his murder, for they know
> Of some most haughty deed or thought
> That waits upon his future days,
> And would through hatred of the bays
> Bring that to nought.

No wonder that a strong ghost is invoked as ally and advocate.

The struggle that each of us necessarily undertakes to deal with our mortality, our freedom, our isolation and our need to make meaning is complicated by our relationships and by the fact that both parties to a relationship face the same set of issues. Each of the four major human concerns that existential psychiatry identifies is ultimately insuperable – we all die, we are all forced to make choices, we all feel our isolation, and we are all required to construct whatever meaning we can from the component parts of our lives. Once a symptom is shared, I become aware that there is an 'other' who is also struggling with his or her heightened version of these concerns.

In childhood, developing awareness of personal identity is followed by the deeper realisation of the separate existence of the other. A sympathetic response is literally a 'gut reaction', and is universal to a greater or lesser degree in relation to someone we love.[8] An empathic response, by contrast, requires a highly developed imaginative capacity, specifically the ability to imagine the experience from the other's point of view. Dylan Thomas responds to his dying father with a desperate plea to 'rage against the dying of the light', but this is surely a reflection of his own existential terror – it is an expression of sympathy, not empathy.

While the Golden Rule expresses the essence of sympathy in 'doing unto others as you would have them do unto you', true empathy can be expressed as 'doing unto others as they would have you do unto them.' Sympathy can actually undermine the sufferer's confidence and well-being if it finds expression in such terms as 'If I were you, (I would fight harder/ignore my symptoms/rush to the doctor, etc.).' An empathic response, on the other hand, provides deep comfort because the 'other' has been able to give accurate expression to the feelings of the sufferer, who now has the reassurance of feeling genuinely understood. As one of Irvin Yalom's patients says, '(Even) though you're alone in your boat, it's always comforting to see the lights of the other boats bobbing nearby'[9] – that is, to see others who know what it's like to be 'alone in your boat.' Depending on the history of a relationship, true empathy can be a difficult and chastening experience. This is probably why it tends to come in 'flashes' of insight, often accompanied by a strong emotional response.

AN EVOLUTIONARY LENS

Chapter 1 acknowledged that it is 'natural' to search for meaning in life, and that this sense of meaning contributes to the elements that make life worth living. We tend to construct a world with ourselves firmly in the middle of the action. Protagoras said that 'Man is the measure of all things, of that which is, that it is and of that which is not, that it is not.' Our foundation myths generally speak of a time when the meaning of existence was self-evident; we were created by god-like creatures of enormous, if not infinite power. We are the children of the divine, 'fallen' from our rightful position in Paradise, seeking to regain our special relationship with a divine creator (or creators) of all things. 'Paradise', literally 'a walled garden', represents our deepest longing for safety, order, beauty and harmony.

In the course of human history, our foundation myths return repeatedly to the idea that we have been cast down from a lofty height, and that somehow we must regain our rightful place. The trajectory of the human race is to have experienced a fall from grace, the depths of human suffering and the restitution of our special privileges (through either individual 'salvation' or the inexorable tide of history). This belief system within the Western tradition is nowhere more evident in the modern world than in the concept of 'American exceptionalism'.[10]

Charles Darwin forced us to consider a radically new way of looking at our place in the world. Perhaps we are not fallen angels after all. Our trajectory is not one of paradise lost and the struggle to return, but of a struggle that began quite literally in the primordial ooze. If we are creatures who have emerged through a process of natural selection, this 'dangerous idea'[11] has innumerable implications for human relationships. What if they have less to do with humans emulating divine love and more to do with perpetuating one's genes, with or without consent? If you help my genes to survive, you make our relationship worth cultivating. If I am related to you, I am more likely to help you to survive.

It is not difficult to understand why humans have so vigorously resisted this insult. If the 'meaning' of life is simply the survival of the fittest genes, then we can radically recast the significance of illness and the role of relationships in the illness experience. These arguments are amusingly pursued in *Madam Bovary's Ovaries, a Darwinian look at literature*.[12] If we are most likely to help those with whom we share the greatest number of genes, Rachel's parents will be the ones to feel the greatest empathy and emotional distress. When the sufferer is not a close relative, illness may make them less attractive because they are less 'fit' from a reproductive perspective – a possibility that Jake clearly fears. Will Carol truly empathise with his problems, or will she seek an alternative partner? On the other hand, if a couple has already formed a close pair bond, and perhaps reproduced together, will this be enough to sustain them when the tide turns from 'the better' to 'the worse'? If we were pushed to make a choice would biology, psychology, philosophy or sociology provide the most coherent account of human behaviour?

SOCIOLOGICAL AND PSYCHOLOGICAL PERSPECTIVES

Although we normally think in terms of biomedical mechanisms (infections, cancer, physical derangements, etc.), Talcott Parsons introduced the idea of illness as medically sanctioned deviant behaviour:

> . . . illness is a state of disturbance in the 'normal' functioning of the total human individual, including both the state of the organism as a biological system and of his personal and social adjustments. It is thus partly biologically and partly socially defined. Participation in the social system is always potentially relevant to the state of illness, to its etiology and to the conditions of successful therapy, as well as to other things.[13]

In this context, 'the sick role' describes the 'personal and social adjustments' that characterise those who claim to be ill. Following Talcott Parsons, Marshall Marinker and others have made a helpful distinction between 'sickness', 'illness' and 'disease.'[14] Marinker described the social element of sickness as follows:

> Sickness is a social role, a status, a negotiated position in the world, a bargain struck between the person henceforward called 'sick', and a society which is prepared to recognise and sustain him.

At the very least, this definition requires that there be at least one 'other' who is willing to accord this status to the sick person.

From a sociological point of view, sick people assume certain social rights and incur certain obligations.[15] First, they are allowed to forego their usual responsibilities in proportion to the type and seriousness of their illness. Although it is usual for a doctor to make the diagnosis that confirms the sick role, the most likely chain of events is that the person who believes him- or herself to be unwell will inform close relatives, friends and/or employers of his or her altered status, and perhaps involve them in the decision to consult a doctor in the first place. This is the stage on which we are concentrating in this consideration of symptoms. It may not be until the next stage that the doctor 'legitimises' the illness and gives advice on precisely how the sick role should be performed (taking time off work or school, going to bed, taking medication, undergoing surgery, etc.).

The second right is the right to be seen as innocent victims of a misfortune, rather than being held responsible for becoming unwell in a way that makes the sufferer feel guilty of some shortcoming.

In exchange for these two rights, the sick have two obligations. The first obligation (in exchange for exemption from normal responsibilities) is to ensure that the illness is not unduly prolonged or manipulated for 'secondary gain.' In other words, the sick person should not become more of a burden on others than is strictly necessary; they should demonstrate a genuine desire to become well again. The second obligation is to seek technically competent help, most commonly by consulting a healthcare provider, and to cooperate in the process of returning to a state of good health.

This is a useful model for considering the social exchanges that occur as soon as symptoms are identified and communicated to others. There are, of course, limits to this model, especially for people like Rachel, Jake and Liz who have chronic or life-threatening illnesses. Other illnesses, such as Jen's, that are associated with lifestyle choices such as smoking, alcohol use or overeating, can involve a measure of blame and social disapproval. This runs counter to the second right that Parsons outlined, of being held to be innocent of blame. Equally threatening to the model is the situation of those who are poor or who live in a remote location from which they may not be able to access appropriate healthcare. Finally, some people may, like Liz, have obligations as single parents, sole breadwinners, small business employers, etc., that force them to keep working even when they should not do so.

Nevertheless, Parsons's model is of interest to us in this situation, because of the idea of a transition from the 'well' role into the sick role. Parsons drew on some of the work of Sigmund Freud to show that humans are subject to drives and desires that may conflict with each other. These potential conflicts are well outlined in our vignettes. Rachel wants to be well, but she would also like to miss violin practice and go to bed, if only her mum could know how bad she feels. Liz is driven to cover up her symptoms, even while she is longing for the 'secondary gain' that might come from asking someone to help her with her burden of sole parenthood. Jake might find Carol reassuringly sympathetic, provided that his illness does not turn her off. If only Jen could tell Geoff about her symptoms, she might finally be able to show him that he is not the only one entitled to assume the sick role.

Freud drew attention to the fact that throughout life people re-apply the characteristic features of individuals with whom they have had significant relationships, in particular the characteristic features of their parents, to others. Although Freud was interested in how such phenomena play out within the therapist–patient relationship,[16] it is easy to see how transference and counter-transference operate within all close relationships, not only in therapeutic settings.

Whenever we think that we might be ill, we have the choice of covering it up and holding fast to the 'well role', or sharing the information with others and tacitly agreeing to enter the 'sick role.' In doing so, we hand over a certain amount of authority to those in whom we confide. Freud's psychoanalytic approach helped to explain why a sick person, or a person who believes that he or she might be sick, might relate to others in particular, sometimes 'uncharacteristic' ways. Illness provides an opportunity to regress. To become unwell is to become vulnerable and potentially dependent. In doing this, we relinquish a certain amount of authority in exchange for care and concern.

The idea of authority appearing in different forms was developed in particular by Max Weber, whose ideas Parsons also considered and incorporated into his own work. Weber argued that we recognise authority in three main guises – rational–legal authority, traditional authority and charismatic authority.[17] Within the period of time before they decide to consult a doctor, a person who is worried about certain symptoms may turn to, and accept, non-medical authority, and especially the traditional authority exerted by family and friends. Obviously Rachel's mum has 'traditional authority', but Geoff probably exerts this kind of authority, too, despite his own illness. Jen certainly seems to accept his right to be very demanding. The power in such relationships may influence the sufferer to seek or avoid medical care, or may lead to conflict if the sufferer and the significant other(s) are at odds about the most appropriate response.

As well as exerting traditional authority, some wise family member or friend, well versed in illness, may also exert 'charismatic authority.' Someone with a strong personality like Carol may eventually persuade a shy person like Jake to do something constructive about his symptoms, even though he would prefer to hide them. She may be able to help him to bridge the gap between his anxieties about his symptoms and sources of help, based on the 'rational–legal authority' vested in medicine.

A number of studies have examined the ways in which children are socialised to react to symptoms. The way in which parents respond to their children's symptoms can reinforce certain beliefs, and the way that parents cope with their own symptoms provides a model that influences later behaviour.[18] For example, Whitehead and colleagues found that childhood reinforcement of cold-illness behaviour significantly predicted adult cold symptoms and disability days, while childhood reinforcement of menstrual illness behaviour significantly predicted adult menstrual symptoms and disability days.

A RELATIONSHIP LENS

At the heart of these existential, evolutionary, psychological and sociological perspectives lies the link between them – the human relationships that are essential for our physical and emotional survival and flourishing.

Each person interprets the altered behaviours of another person in the light of their relationship status and in the light of their own personality and past experiences. It may take time to realise that a previously healthy individual is manifesting the first symptoms of illness, or that a person with previously controlled symptoms is experiencing an exacerbation.

The people who are closest to the potential patients do not yet consider seriously the possibility that Rachel, Jake, Liz or Jen may be ill. There are other possible explanations that have nothing to do with health and illness. Rachel may simply be recalcitrant, Jake may be shy, and Liz and Jen may be overworked. Admittedly, Rachel's mother is tuned in to the possibility of illness ('You seem a bit peaky. What's up?'), but she is soon distracted by other responsibilities.

Rachel's mother has a direct responsibility for her daughter's well-being, particularly since she is the person in the family who sees Rachel most often, and is most likely to notice whether her behaviour is unusual. Liz's status as a single mother gives her an even more significant responsibility to protect her daughter from any adverse effects that might arise from her own epilepsy. Sophie herself remains unaware of her mother's precarious position, simply because Liz protects her from worry by covering up her symptoms.

Jake and Carol share a different kind of relationship, one that does not carry with it the same burden of direct responsibility that a parent carries for a child. They are two young adults whose relationship may progress or falter at this early stage. If Carol realises that Jake has a number of health problems, this may influence her to terminate the relationship. Later, if the relationship becomes more firmly established, she may find it easier to take such health problems in her stride. Geoff and Jen have a long-standing relationship, but the effects of Geoff's stroke will have changed the dynamic – and Jen's possibly serious diagnosis may change it even more.

Rachel's mother may be angry when she discovers that her daughter has put herself in danger by failing to disclose symptoms that carry such serious implications. She is likely to experience guilt ('Why did she feel unable to tell me?') and may even face this question from Rachel's father or other family members. This in turn may translate into overly solicitous concern as Rachel's symptoms are being investigated. One or both parents may become excessively protective, and may worry when Rachel is out of contact – for example, at school. If insulin-dependent diabetes is confirmed, the need to notify Rachel's school about her condition may cause conflict if Rachel wants to hide her problem from teachers and friends.

Alex and Rachel have a relationship that is fairly typical of adolescent boys and younger sisters – frequent arguments and mutual irritation. However, when a crisis such as a serious illness occurs, siblings may find it difficult to express their underlying affection and concern, resulting in behaviour that is seen by adults as inappropriate ('Can't you see that your sister isn't well?'). Rachel's problem may even lead to an exaggeration of their usual squabbling. Her symptoms are a reminder to Alex that he is also vulnerable – a most unwelcome concept for an adolescent boy who is fantasising about his unlimited powers and immortality. Because adolescence is often a time of heightened existential concerns, it can be especially difficult to face the fact that one is powerless to prevent bad things from happening to those whom one loves. (The dramatic potential of this dilemma helps to explain the popular appeal of Morris Gleitzman's play for children, *Two Weeks with the Queen*.[19])

Rachel's symptoms are likely to occupy her parents' attention for some time, and Alex may find this difficult, especially if his parents seem to be distracted and less available to him in both emotional and practical terms ('So, who's coming to see my soccer game?'). If he expresses resentment, his behaviour may be construed as selfishness and lead his parents to develop a more 'black-and-white' view of their children. Given that Rachel's mother may already be experiencing guilt, Alex could become a convenient scapegoat, distracting her from her own perceived failure.

In Jake's case, his relationship with Carol is still in a formative stage, and neither of them can presume too much about the other or about the relationship. Jake's gastrointestinal symptoms are likely to be mainly psychological in origin, as evidenced by his response to Carol's sudden appearance at his flat. The fact that she is willing to take the initiative in turning up uninvited at his flat suggests that she is unlikely to be discouraged by his problem. In fact her behaviour suggests a 'can do' attitude that Jake may find very reassuring. After all, if Carol can accept his problem without undue fuss, perhaps he can also trust her to understand how he feels about having psoriasis as well. So long as she does not appear to trivialise his concerns, Carol is likely to have a very positive influence on Jake's self-esteem by helping him to normalise his experience.

RESPONSIBILITY TO THE SUFFERING

The obligation of parents towards their children, so poignantly described in Yeats' poem, is powerfully supported by biological, psychological and social impulses. Rachel's parents will not hesitate to seek help on her behalf.

Similarly, Liz, as a sole parent, has a duty to seek medical help so that she can continue to care for Sophie. When symptoms appear in a child, parents confront the possibility of a terrible loss if the symptoms are sinister. They become aware, perhaps for the first time, of their full parental investment. When a child becomes gravely ill, parents mourn not only the loss of present well-being, but also their fantasies of a perfect future.

For adults, different issues emerge. A couple like Geoff and Jen confronts the emergence of symptoms in one of the pair. In most societies, some version of the principle that one makes a pair-bond commitment 'for better, for worse' prevails. This principle can be severely tested by symptoms of serious debilitating (or potentially fatal) diseases or injury. Those who may find themselves responsible for the care of another are likely to look ahead with some anxiety to consider the impact on their own life and the adjustments that may be necessary – in particular the time required for visits to doctors and other healthcare providers, and for tests and special treatments.

As well as adjusting to the practical implications of symptoms that turn out to be portents of serious illness, the potential carer may need to make aesthetic adjustments. A partner who was chosen for their physical attractiveness may now seem flawed and imperfect. A partner who was seen as strong and caring may become less potent and more needy. These changes test the basis of relationships, and can reveal influences that were not previously recognised as significant. The man who has relied on his partner's resourcefulness may find himself resenting her inability to continue in this role. A woman who has acted as family peacemaker may find that simmering resentments surface when she is unable to keep conflict at bay. A couple planning their retirement may find that the possibility of a serious illness that affects the wife unmasks their shared expectation that the husband would be the first to fall ill and that his wife would outlive him.

Symptoms can strip away our belief in our invulnerability. When they occur in another, symptoms can remind us of how we really feel about them and about ourselves. With understated emotion, here is another of Yeats' poems, this one for Lady Gregory – *A Friend's Illness*:

> Sickness brought me this
> Thought, in that scale of his:
> Why should I be dismayed
> Though flame had burned the whole
> World, as it were a coal,
> Now I have seen it weighed
> Against a soul?

REFERENCES

1 Yeats WB (Finneran RJ, editor). *The Collected Poems of WB Yeats: revised second edition.* New York: Simon and Schuster; 1996.

2 Office for National Statistics. *Mortality Statistics Series. Infant mortality rates by sex, England and Wales, 1928–98.* Newport: Office for National Statistics; Series DH1, no.30. London: TSO; 1999.

3 Mystakidou K, Parpa E *et al.* Cancer information disclosure in different cultural contexts. *Support Care Cancer.* 2004; **12:** 147–54.

4 Fromm E. *The Fear of Freedom.* London: Routledge & Kegan Paul; 1942.

5 Sartre J-P (Barnes HE, trans.). *Existential Psychoanalysis.* Chicago: Henry Regnery Co; 1962.

6 Yalom ID. *Existential Psychotherapy.* New York: Basic Books; 1980.

7 Andrews G, Page AC. Outcome measurement, outcome management and monitoring. *Aust N Z J Psychiatry.* 2005; **39:** 649–51.

8 Greenspan SI, Benderly BL. *The Growth of the Mind and the Endangered Origins of Intelligence.* Cambridge, MA: Perseus Books; 1997.

9 Yalom ID. *Love's Executioner.* New York: Basic Books; 1989.

10 Weaver J. Original simplicities and present complexities: Reinhold Niebuhr, ethnocentrism, and the myth of American exceptionalism. *J Am Acad Relig.* **63:** 231–48.

11 Dennett D. *Darwin's Dangerous Idea.* New York: Simon & Schuster; 1995.

12 Barasch DP, Barasch NR. *Madame Bovary's Ovaries: a Darwinian look at literature.* New York: Delacorte Press; 2005.

13 Parsons T. Social structure and dynamic process: the case of modern medical practice. In: *The Social System.* London: RKP; 1951.

14 Marinker M. Why make people patients? *J Med Ethics.* 1975; **1:** 81–4.

15 Cockerham WC. *Medical Sociology.* 8th ed. Englewood Cliffs, NJ: Prentice Hall; 2001. pp. 156–78.

16 Freud S. The dynamics of transference. In: *The Standard Edition of the Complete Psychological Works of Sigmund Freud. Vol XII (1911–1913)* (Trans. J Strachey). London: The Hogarth Press; 1958, pp. 97–109.

17 Elwell F. *The Sociology of Max Weber;* www.faculty.rsu.edu/~felwell/Theorists/Weber/Whome.htm (accessed 4 January 2006).

18 Whitehead WE, Crowell MD, Heller BR *et al.* Modeling and reinforcement of the sick role during childhood predicts adult illness behavior. *Psychosom Med.* 1994; **56:** 541–50.

19 Gleitzman M. *Two Weeks with the Queen.* London: Puffin Books; 1999.

CHAPTER 7

Another day with a headache: semiotics of everyday symptoms

RAIMO PUUSTINEN

In medical literature, the words 'sign' and 'symptom' commonly occur as twinned terms when a particular disease is discussed. 'Symptom' is commonly defined as a subjective phenomenon, something causing 'concern to the patient', while 'sign' refers to the 'objective and verifiable mark of disease' representing a 'solid, indisputable fact', to quote an eminent textbook of internal medicine.[1]

As straightforward as the use of the terms 'sign' and 'symptom' in medicine may seem, there are numerous theoretical and practical problems interwoven in the setting. In this chapter I shall examine the meaning of 'symptom' in relation to 'sign' from a semiotic viewpoint, together with its implications for medical theory and practice.

FEELING ILL

We started this book with four short stories depicting how pain and illness interfere with people's everyday lives. In the first story, something in the way that Rachel is behaving attracts her mother's attention. She looks at her daughter and says that the girl seems to be 'a bit peaky.' Rachel says she is tired of playing the violin. But there seems to be more to it, since she also says she wants to go to bed and that she is fed up, exhausted and starving. 'Being peaky' is now expanding to include other phenomena, but it does not yet form a comprehensive picture to the mother – the girl can't be starving, as she has just eaten a whole packet of biscuits.

Rachel is just as confused by what is going on. She feels thirsty, but drinking does not take away the thirst. And she has been running to the toilet for weeks. She also recognises various other bodily sensations, such as shivering and sweating, feeling sick, cold and dizzy, and being too tired to move. There is obviously something wrong with her, but none of the people in the story can understand what it is.

In the second story, Jake has a problem with his skin, diagnosed as psoriasis. Because of the way he looks, he excludes himself from others by living alone, not showing his bare skin publicly, and refusing to engage in intimate relationships.

However, his problem is not just the skin but also his bowel. It lets him down more and more often, so that he needs to rush to a toilet even in intimate moments. He attributes this to greasy food and stress. But why should they cause problems like this? All he knows is that the abdominal cramps are indicating that in a few moments he will need to go to the bathroom, quickly.

In our third story, Liz has epilepsy, which was diagnosed in childhood. Now she is having a headache, which has sometimes precipitated an epileptic attack. However, there is no sensation of aura today. She has had the headache since the morning, but there seems to be nothing unusual about it. Her headache is, for her, a sign of stress, and the lack of another sign, the aura, indicates that there is no epileptic fit to be expected.

In the fourth story, Jen is taking care of her husband, who has suffered a stroke. She has visited a doctor because of her persistent cough and traces of blood in her morning sputum. The doctor has suggested further investigations in a clinic. When she receives a letter from the Royal Infirmary, the unopened envelope carries meanings so heavy that her knees grow weak.

In these stories we find people having to cope with various ailments and worries. Some of their problems have been medically diagnosed, such as psoriasis and epilepsy, but many of their symptoms lack an explanation as yet. They are just feeling ill. However, even in these short fragments we notice that the terms 'symptom' and 'sign' seem to carry different meanings in people's lives compared with their meaning in a medical vocabulary. What we call in medicine a symptom can be a sign for the person that there is something wrong with their bodily or mental functions. In order to understand better the usage of the terms 'sign' and 'symptom' in medicine, we need first to discuss the concept of 'sign' in general.

SIGNS

A sign is commonly defined as something that refers to something else. A red light on a car's dashboard is a sign that the car is running out of fuel. A bell ringing in a school playground is a sign that it is time to get back to class. A certain kind of rash on a child's skin is a sign that the child has measles.

A somewhat more elaborate definition of a sign describes it as a 'semiotic entity consisting of a sign vehicle connected with meaning.'[2] A sign thus consists of two aspects. A vehicle such as a raised index finger, connected to meaning – for example, when it is raised in a pub – is a sign, in this case to the bartender that it is a time for another pint. However, the same raised index finger at an auction carries a different meaning from that in a bar. A red light on a car's dashboard is different from a red light at a traffic light. A bell ringing in a school playground has a different meaning from a bell ringing on one's bedroom table. How then does a gesture, a colour or a sound cease to be just a gesture, a colour or a sound and become connected to and be a conveyor of different meanings in different settings?

This problem has intrigued philosophers since antiquity, but the systematic study of signs, or semiotics as it is now commonly called, has developed to its present form only since the late nineteenth century. The term 'semiotic' was introduced in 1689 by John Locke, who proposed in his *Essay Concerning Human Understanding* a division of the sciences into natural philosophy, ethics and semiotics. Locke defined semiotics as 'logic the business whereof is to consider the nature of signs, the mind makes use for the understanding of things, or conveying its knowledge to others.'[3]

During the last few decades, semiotics has grown into a vast discipline contributing especially to the study of signs and sign systems in language, culture, cybernetics, biology and medicine.

SEMIOTICS AND MEDICINE

Medicine deals with signs and symptoms. Their nature and mutual relationship has been a central problem in medicine since the advent of medical theory. The author of a Hippocratic treatise that was compiled more than two millennia ago discusses the question of interpreting patients' signs and symptoms as follows:

> [The] physician must have recourse to reasoning from the symptoms with which he is presented . . . the symptoms which patients . . . describe to their physician are based on guesses about a possible cause rather than knowledge about it. . . . When the physician cannot make an exact diagnosis from the

patient's description of his symptoms, the doctor must employ other methods for his guidance. . . . By weighing up the significance of . . . various (bodily) signs it is possible to deduce of what disease they are the result. . . . Even when nature herself does not produce such signs, they may be revealed by certain harmless measures known to those practised in the science.[4]

This short paragraph addresses the same problems that we also encounter in modern medicine when we try to understand our patients' complaints. The ancient author suggests, first, that a physician may reach a diagnosis on the basis of the patient's symptoms alone, but often he needs to deduce the disease 'by weighing up the significance of various signs.'

In our patient stories, Rachel's symptoms lead a physician to consider the possibility of a case of juvenile diabetes. The appearance of Jake's skin has, in turn, led the examining physician to deduce a diagnosis of psoriasis, while Liz's concurrent seizures have been weighed as a sign of the illness we call epilepsy. Medical diagnosis can thus be considered to be an act of inference – that is, organisation, categorisation and deduction from the patient's symptoms and signs to medical concepts.

In contemporary semiotics there are three main theoretical approaches to the problem of signs – dyadic, triadic and dialogic. In what follows I shall consider them in relation to medical theory and practice.

The dyadic sign

The Swiss linguist Ferdinand Saussure (1857–1913) proposed a dyadic theory of signs where a sign consists of two components, the signifier (*signifiant*) and the signified (*signifié*).[5] A signifier is the material form that a sign has. This may be a word appearing as a composition of sounds (e.g. p-s-o-r-i-a-s-i-s). A signifier refers to something signified, and what is signified is a concept (rather than a substantive instance of the concept), in this case a concept of a certain medical category. That is, according to Saussure's theory a sign does not refer directly to an object itself, such as Jake's affected skin, but to an *idea* cast in a concept referring to that particular type of skin condition.

For Saussure, a sign, as exemplified in a word, has meaning only in the context of other signs – that is, other words. Meaning is a relational phenomenon in a dyadic signifier–signified referential system. Both signifier and signified are products of cultural conventions. This is typified in the way that we create and use words in different languages, where different words stand for similar concepts. For example, 'fever' in English, '*fiévre*' in French and '*Fieber*' in German all refer to the concept of raised body temperature.

Because Saussure was first and foremost a linguist, his semiotic theory, or *sémiologie* as he called it, is grounded in language in relation to meaning in a cultural context. As a consequence, his theory has had strong influence not only on linguistics but also on cultural studies.

However, the problem of sign and symptom in medicine seems to be more complicated than a simple dyadic relationship between a particular sound composition and a particular concept (such as that of a medical diagnosis). The author of the Hippocratic quotation above writes that 'the symptoms which patients describe to their physician are based on guesses about a possible cause rather than knowledge about it.' It seems, then, that in order to gain a fuller understanding of the patient's complaints we need to expand our treatment of a sign in medicine with a third element, namely the pre-existing knowledge against which signs and symptoms are interpreted.

The triadic sign

The American philosopher Charles Sanders Peirce (1839–1914) proposed a triadic definition of the word 'sign', where a sign is composed of three components, a *representamen*, an *object* and an *interpretant*. The representamen is the material form of a sign which refers to an object; for a traffic signal, the red light is the representamen, referring to the imperative to stop. Note that the *object* here is not a material object but an intentional object – the state of affairs to which the sign points. The interpretant is the process of thought by which the sign gains meaning (*see* Endnote [a]). For instance, it is evaluated against a pre-existing system of signs, in this case the system of signs comprising knowledge of traffic rules and regulations.[6]

Every sign is thus devoid of meaning until it is interpreted by a subsequent thought, an interpretant. In fact, a sign is not a sign at all without it. A red light at a traffic light is not a sign for a person who has no idea of the way that modern traffic is organised. For him or her there is just a post with a red light. It conveys no meaning – that is, it does not refer to anything beyond itself.

The formation and interpretation of a sign is an active and continuous process. We can see this in our case stories, where all of the characters are trying to fit the phenomena they encounter to their pre-existing knowledge about the world. Jake is trying to explain his bowel symptoms as being caused by greasy food and stress. Liz deals with her symptoms in her own semiotic system, or *semiosphere* as we may call it, where her headache acts as a representamen (signifier), her stress is the sign's object (signified), and her knowledge of the nature of epilepsy is the interpretant against which the headache is evaluated and given meaning.

For Jen, her cough, bloodstained sputum and weight loss, and her knowledge of the possibility of tuberculosis, together constitute a meaning so burdensome that it makes her physically weak. However, in the case of Rachel, neither she nor her mother can make sense of the phenomena that they encounter, since they are not yet able to fit them to any pre-existing knowledge.

A commonplace clinical example of how an interpretant is necessary for sign formation in medicine is an interpretation of a chest X-ray image. Where a layman sees just random shades of grey, a radiologist may discern signs indicating a possibility of, say, a case of pneumonia. To form this interpretation, the radiologist weighs their knowledge of the patient's condition against their pre-existing knowledge of the various ways in which pneumonia may manifest itself in a chest X-ray (*see* Endnote [b]). (This also exemplifies the fact that the interpretation of the patient's signs and symptoms in medicine is not based on passive observation, but is an active and continuous process following the course of the patient's illness.)

It seems, then, that Peirce's triadic approach to the problem of a sign applies to medicine better than does Saussure's dyadic model. However, we need to take the question of signification in medicine still further. The diagnostic and therapeutic process in medicine rests fundamentally on doctor–patient communication. Yet it is noteworthy that in the Hippocratic quotation cited above there is no account of the way in which the doctor communicates with his patient. Curiously, this is the case throughout the Hippocratic corpus. (*See* Endnote [c].) The author notes, briefly, that if the doctor cannot deduce the diagnosis from what the patient presents, he 'must employ other methods for his guidance.' As we saw, the signs needed to establish a diagnosis 'may be revealed by certain harmless measures known to those practised in the science.' Here the patient appears to be merely a passive informant, and if he or she does not provide enough information, the physician needs to look for more. However, in our stories the patients are not only reporting their symptoms. They are also involved in continuous dialogues (both internal and external) when trying to make sense of the nature of their problems. This is also the case in all of the medical encounters where the physician engages in a dialogue with his or her patient. Even in cases where the patient is for some reason not able to talk, there is usually someone with the patient with whom the physician initiates a conversation. How can this necessary condition of medicine be addressed with semiotic theory?

Dialogic sign

The Russian philosopher of language, Valentin Voloshinov (1895–1936), introduced a theory of signs whereby signs emerge and are formed within inter-individual communication through physical means such as gestures, expressions, voices, intonations, etc. In this process anything at all has the potential to mediate meaning – that is, to be a sign. The nature of the sign materialises in, and is determined by, communication.[7]

For Voloshinov, the spoken word is a sign *par excellence*. Yet a word as a physical sound composition has no meaning by itself. It acquires meaning only through social interaction. Through this interaction a word not only becomes a mediator of interpersonal communication, but also acts as a mediator of the individual's inner communication, his inner speech. Our thoughts are mediated by words, and the act of thinking can be considered, essentially, as an act of an inner dialogue.[7]

To illustrate this with a clinical example, let us picture a person whose primary response to a damaging event, such as stepping barefoot on a piece of broken glass, may be just an abrupt change of his physical posture. This is a purely a motor response and it contains no meaning. However, as soon as it becomes conscious it becomes a subject of *inner* dialogue ('What . . .?'). This inner dialogue is conceptualised with the words of internal utterance, and it creates meaning through a dialogic question–answer analysis of the possible cause of the pain.[8]

This inner process can be seen in each of our case stories. Rachel has a continuous inner dialogue with herself when she tries to make sense of her discomfort. 'That was the funny thing', she relates, when after drinking a glass of water she is even thirstier, and can remember no time recently when she was not thirsty. 'No! Not again. Not now!', Jake cries silently when the cramps start. Liz engages in an inner dialogue with her absent mother: '*When you're feeling that way*,' she could hear her mother hectoring, '*Sit down or lie down. Lying is better. If you can*.' And Jen asks herself 'What if it was TB? What then?'

Our characters are also involved with outer dialogues when trying to understand their sensations. Rachel and her mother develop a dialogue that seems to lead nowhere in terms of understanding of what is going on. Jake's elderly co-worker initiates a discussion when he notices how Jake's psoriasis is affecting his whole life. When he utters the word 'psoriasis' the young man blushes. Thus a mere sound composition carries meaning between the two, causing a visible physical response in Jake's body. And when the young man is trying to cope with his abdominal cramps, Carol addresses his behaviour by saying that if she hadn't known better she would think that she wasn't welcome. While Jake cannot find words to reply, Carol answers herself by saying 'I know better. Come here, you daft thing. *Now*.'

Liz is also involved in a continuous dialogue (internal and external) while trying to put her headache into context. She goes through the events of the day and ends up blaming herself. When her daughter notices there is something wrong with her mother, they engage in a dialogue as they try to find a meaning for what is going on. When the girl asks her mother if she is all right, Liz replies that she is fine. The girl does not accept this since, to her, Liz does not look fine at all. Liz solves the problem by attributing her headache to the weather, and tries to change the subject. However, her inner dialogue keeps on going, and expands to involve a number of other people, such as her mother, the nurse, Carlos, his lawyer and, again, her daughter. The symptom has not merely initiated a dialogue with her daughter, but has expanded to an inner conversation with individuals who are connected in one way or another to her life and well-being. And finally, Jen has been negotiating her symptoms with a doctor, who is suggesting further examinations at a clinic, and insisting that she needs to discuss the situation with her husband.

To summarise, all of the above three semiotic approaches can be applied, to an extent, to the analysis of signs in medicine. Since Voloshinov founds his semiotics upon human communication – a fundamental activity for medical practice – it is his theory that I shall apply in exploring the nature of symptoms further below.

THE SYMPTOM AS A SIGN

While in medical vocabulary the terms 'sign' and 'symptom' are considered to be essentially separate entities, a symptom as a subjective experience is also a sign for the person who has it. For a patient a symptom is, as Baer expresses it, a 'sign with special communicative powers. There is no sign to match it in existential value and depth.'[9]

Following Voloshinov's semiotics, the meaning that a symptom gains as a sign is developed by the dialogue that it initiates. A symptom as a subjective experience may arouse an inner dialogue ('*What . . .?*'), but it can also become outwardly orientated and initiate a whole set of discussions with a variety of people involved in the person's life, as we see in our case stories.

When a person communicates their symptoms, they borrow the words from the stock of available signs – that is, language. The utterance and its interpretation are modified by the reciprocal relationship between the speaker and the listener. The immediate social situation and the broader social milieu determine the resulting structure and contents of the dialogue which defines the modes and realms of potential inferences – be that bad behaviour, greasy food, stress or any other explanation available for the participants in the dialogue. And there is nothing to be gained outside these realms so long as no other actor participates in the dialogic event.

If the inferences that are generated and mediated by the dialogic process (internal or external) do not lead to a satisfactory solution for the problem of the symptom as a sign, the afflicted person may seek assistance in whatever forms it may be available in their community. If the person reaches for a professional interpretation, be it from an indigenous healer or a local GP, he moves from one *semiosphere* to another. He departs from his private semiosphere (which may include those people closest to him) and moves to the public semiosphere, to what the community in general considers to be possible modes of interpretation for the person's symptom.

In the end, the whole route from a response-arousing event, through the experience of it conceptualised and expressed in internal and external dialogue, to the shared understanding, to a possible decision to seek professional advice, through the process of a professional consultation and, finally, to the diagnosis and the therapeutic process, lies entirely across social territory and is mediated with signs. Therefore the form of an illness process from its beginning to its very end is culturally shaped and restricted in its realms of potential expressions existing in this particular (sub)culture.

TRANSFORMING A SYMPTOM

If the person decides to consult a physician because of a symptom, the doctor's task is to translate the patient's presentation of symptoms into medical terms, and to construct the diagnosis on the basis of the information acquired. The act of understanding is thus a response. It translates what is being understood into a new context from which a response can be made. The patient's expression, 'I am always tired,' 'I have pain,' 'I feel dizzy' must be understood and translated into the concepts that the physician uses in his or her diagnostic and therapeutic thinking.

In medical examination, the eliciting of symptoms and production of signs take place through the method of questioning. Observation is always an answer to a question. The choice of questions and observations made is restricted to the concepts applied in the process of examination. The answer to a question has to be formulated in terms of the same concepts as those in which the question itself was formulated.[10]

Every discipline, including medicine, possesses its own conceptual material and formulates the signs specific to itself. Thus a sign is created by and for some specific function, and it remains inseparable from it. However, no sign, once taken in and given meaning, remains in isolation. The understanding of any sign is tied to the situation in which the sign is implemented, and this is always a *social* situation. In the process of understanding symptoms and signs we relate our experience to a context made up of other signs with which we are familiar. Therefore no matter how objective a biological event it may refer to, a medical sign (be it a palpable mass, a laboratory reading or a shadow in a chest X-ray) can be understood only with the help of other signs.

Medical signs are created on the basis of the ontological model of health and illness that the physician applies in their practice. However, a medical sign is not a passively existing fact that is merely waiting to be noticed by the physician. It is a product of active inquiry and of a set of procedures performed by the physician along those lines of reasoning that guide their thinking, as the author of the Hippocratic treatise quoted above also maintains. For example, a modern physician is not concerned about the possibility of, say, an evil eye causing the patient's problems. Thus he will not attempt to look for or produce signs that indicate its presence. A physician follows the logic of the current medical theory where the essence of disease is tied to the events and derangements within the patient's body (psychiatric phenomena partly excluded).

Medicine holds scientific objectivity as an ideal for its practice. Yet in everyday medical practice the 'contextuality' of the medical encounter cannot be avoided. This contextuality modifies the dialogue between the doctor and the patient. For example, in a busy emergency clinic the focus is on the most urgent matters in the patient's condition, and the dialogue between the patient and the physician may be restricted to just a few questions and answers. However, even when the situation favours an unhurried medical interview, as in a quiet country GP's surgery, patients do not automatically report all of their symptoms, nor are all of the potential medical signs necessarily produced and observed. If the patient is not willing or able to disclose all of their symptoms, and if the physician does not ask appropriate questions, or if he or she fails to pay attention to the verbal or non-verbal cues that the patient presents, some of the patient's ailments may never be reported or noticed. The diagnosis is thus a result of an interpersonal interaction and the intentional production of a *set* of signs.

To sum up, the translation of the patient's symptoms into medical signs, as with any other sign-phenomenon, is a social process. Its specificity consists in its being located between individuals, and in its being the medium of their communication. What is created, what symptoms are brought into the dialogue and what signs are formed during the process of medical examination are determined by the very nature of this particular and always unique encounter between a physician and his or her patient. And it is precisely here that the variability of different doctor–patient encounters – and the possibility of diagnostic error and various forms of mis-readings and discontent among the participants in this dialogic event – become comprehensible.

SYMPTOMS WITHOUT A DISEASE

It is fairly common for a patient to present with symptoms that the examining physician is unable to connect to any diagnostic category used in contemporary medical theory.[11] This may be due to any of at least three reasons. First, perhaps the patient does not have a disease, but they are just worried that some everyday phenomenon, such as fatigue, flatulence or itching, may indicate a medical condition that requires diagnosis and treatment. Secondly, perhaps the physician's failure to establish a diagnosis may be due to professional incompetence. That is, the signs are there but the physician is not able to produce (elicit) them. Thirdly, perhaps the patient does have a disease, but contemporary medical theory does not yet recognise the condition as a separate disease entity. In all of these cases the patient may end up in a vicious circle of consulting an increasing number of specialists in the hope of finding an explanation for their troublesome symptoms.

To overcome the problem of symptoms without a recognisable disease, contemporary medical theory has gathered different sets of symptoms under such labels as, for example, 'chronic fatigue syndrome', 'fibromyalgia' or 'repetitive strain injury', in the hope of finding strategies for physicians to cope with these patients[12] and, eventually, plausible medical explanations and treatments for their ailments.[13]

Another approach in current medical practice is to treat medically unexplained symptoms as an indication of an underlying psychiatric condition, such as depression or anxiety. Such patients can also be seen as suffering from a so-called somatisation disorder. In this case it is assumed that the psychiatric condition manifests itself through bodily symptoms, while there is nothing wrong with the patient's body.[14] However, addressing the problem of a symptom without a medical sign in more depth is beyond the scope of this essay. This question will be discussed more thoroughly in a later volume of this series.

SYMPTOM AND MEANING

When a symptom does fall within an established medical category, its meaning is not thereby exhausted. When we are ill, our symptoms, as well as interrupting our daily life, may call into question our whole existence. Shortness of breath can make us terrified of dying. A severe headache can make us cancel a meeting no matter how important it may be. A chronic bowel irritation may lead us to adjust our life according to the location of the nearest public lavatory.

We can see in all of our case stories how the characters' symptoms penetrate their daily lives and carry meanings that concern their whole being in the world.

This seems to have been the case since the very first documentation of human health, illness and suffering. For example, the Bible depicts how Job is afflicted with various pains and sufferings. However, he did not deal with his symptoms merely as a medical problem (in fact, he cursed physicians for being worthless liars[15]), but saw his torment in the context of his relationship with God. This relationship is made visible through numerous dialogues between Job and his family and friends and, eventually, with God himself. Through these dialogues a new meaning is generated and Job is, in the end, freed from his agonies.

To take another example from world literature, in his short story *A Case History*, Anton Chekhov depicts how a young girl was suffering from palpitations so severe that they kept her awake at night and caused the whole household to be terrified that she would die. Several doctors had been consulted, and they had all agreed that the problem was in the girl's nerves, but the condition was benign and there should have been nothing to worry about. However, this explanation, and the medications prescribed, had not freed the girl from her misery. Her symptoms persisted and they were driving the family to despair. Then a certain young doctor entered the scene and was able to see the girl's symptoms not just in the context of her body but also in the historical and social circumstances in which she lived. This opened up the possibility of a dialogue with the girl, offering new meanings for her symptoms that might, eventually, help her to find a cure for her misery.[16]

It seems then that a symptom, even when explained medically, inevitably becomes filled with meanings that extend well beyond what is expressed in medical vocabulary. The meaning that a symptom gains is not just personal and atomistic. It is derived from the cultural realms in which the afflicted person lives, and its use aims to make sense of their pains and ailments. Therefore the ways in which we reason about (and from) our symptoms vary according to time and place, no matter how similar the events in our bodies may seem from a medical point of view. Had the individuals in our case stories lived in another era or culture, the discussions and meanings generated would have found other forms and contents. Acknowledging that our interpretations of symptoms are socially developed and determined, it becomes possible to study them not only as medical phenomena but also as cultural ones. This approach has been successfully adopted by medical an-thropologists,[17-19] but despite the conceptual tools offered by semiotics only a few attempts have been made to address the problem of the symptom in the clinical context.[8,9,20,21] Adopting semiotic methods for analysing the pathway from a symptom to a medical diagnosis (or a lack of it) could help us to gain a deeper understanding of our everyday symptoms and their relationship to current medical theory and practice.

ENDNOTES

[a] Peirce's notion of 'interpretant' is somewhat ambiguous, since he is not always clear about this concept. I shall rely here on the definition of the 'interpretant' that Peirce gives in a letter to William James: '. . . if the Sign be the sentence "Hamlet was mad", to understand what this means one must know that men are sometimes in that strange state; one must have seen madmen or read about them; and it will be all the better if one specifically knows . . . what Shakespeare's notion of insanity was . . . to put together the different subjects as the sign represents them as related – that is the main of the Interpretant-forming . . . the Interpretant of the sign (is) – its 'significance'.[22] (Peirce distinguishes in his writings different types of interpretants, but that discussion is beyond the scope of this essay.)

[b] It is noteworthy that Russian radiologists use the term 'semiotics' when referring to the interpretation of radiological findings, while in the French medical literature the term 'semiology' is used to interpret medical signs in general.

[c] This observation is based on the material available in the collection of Hippocratic texts in the Loeb Classical Library Volumes I–VIII, Harvard University Press.

REFERENCES

1 Isselbacher K, Martin J, editors. *Harrison's Principles of Internal Medicine*. 13th ed. Tokyo: McGraw-Hill; 1994. p. 2.

2 Nöth W. *Handbook of Semiotics*. Bloomington, IN: Indiana University Press; 1995. p. 79.

3 Locke J. *An Essay Concerning Human Understanding, Volume II*. Whitefish, MT: Kessinger Publishing; 2004 (originally published in 1689), p. 272.

4 Lloyd GER, editor. *Hippocratic Writings*. Harmondsworth: Penguin Books; 1983. pp. 145–7.

5 Saussure F. *Course in General Linguistics*. Chicago, IL: Open Court Publishing Company; 2000. pp. 65–9.

6 Hoopes J, editor. *Peirce on Signs. Writings on semiotic by Charles Sanders Peirce*. Chapel Hill, NC: The University of North Carolina Press; 1991. pp. 8–13.

7 Voloshinov VN. *Marxism and the Philosophy of Language*. Cambridge, MA: Harvard University Press; 1993. pp. 8–14.

8 Puustinen R. Bakhtin's philosophy and medical practice: toward a semiotic theory of doctor–patient interaction. *Med Health Care Philos*. 1999; **2**: 275–81.

9 Baer E. *Medical Semiotics*. Lanham, MD: University Press of America; 1988.

10 Hintikka J, Hintikka MB. Sherlock Holmes confronts modern logic: toward a theory of information-seeking through questioning. In: Eco U, Sebeok TA, editors. *The Sign of Three: Dupin, Holmes, Peirce*. Bloomington, IN: Indiana University Press; 1983.

11 Weijden T, Velsen M, Dinant G-J *et al.* Unexplained complaints in general practice: prevalence, patients' expectations, and professionals' test-ordering behavior. *Med Decision Making*. 2003; **23**: 226–31.

12 Malterud K. Symptoms as a source of medical knowledge: understanding medically unexplained disorders in women. *Fam Med*. 2000; **32**: 603–11.

13 Quintner J, Buchanan D, Cohen M *et al.* Signification and pain: a semiotic reading of fibromyalgia. *Theor Med Bioethics*. 2003; **24**: 345–54.

14 De Waal M, Arnold I, Eekhof A. Somatoform disorders in general practice. *Br J Psychiatry.* 2004; **184:** 470–6.

15 *Job 13: 3–5.*

16 Puustinen R. Voices to be heard: the many positions of a physician in Anton Chekhov's short story, *A Case History. J Med Ethics Med Humanities.* 2000; **1:** 37–42.

17 Kleinman A. *Patients and Healers in the Context of Culture.* Berkeley, CA: University of California Press; 1981.

18 Good B. *Medicine, Rationality and Experience: an anthropological perspective.* Cambridge: Cambridge University Press; 1996.

19 Martinez-Hernandez A. *What's Behind the Symptom?* Singapore: Harwood Academic Publishers; 2000.

20 Staiano K. *Interpreting Signs of Illness: a case study in medical semiotics.* Berlin: Mouton de Gruyter; 1986.

21 Nessa J. About signs and symptoms: can semiotics expand the view of clinical medicine? *Theor Med Bioethics.* 1996; **17:** 363–77.

22 Peirce C. A letter to William James, EP. 1909; **2:** 493–4. In: *The Commens Dictionary of Peirce's Terms;* www.helsinki.fi/science/commens/dictionary.html (entry: interpretant).

CHAPTER 8

Giving meaning to symptoms

ROLF AHLZÉN

It is often asserted that life has to have a meaning. To look for a meaning in events or phenomena seems to be an essential part of what it is to be a human being. The opposite of 'meaningful' – devoid of meaning, meaningless – has strong negative associations. A life without meaning is absurd. We are used to thinking that all people, at least if they are true to their authentic selves, search for meaning in their lives – and that this is a strong force behind their actions. Meaning, in this sense, is what makes life worth living. If this is so, why then is meaning such an elusive concept? Or, to play a little with the word, what is really the meaning of using such an enigmatic concept as 'meaning'?

Meaning is certainly not always a concept that is intended to capture our entire sense of life. It is used in a bewildering number of contexts. The meaning of a word as a linguistic category is certainly not similar to the meaning of my whole existence. The meaning of a question seems to be its point – 'what it is seeking after.' The function of any sign, as semiotics tells us, is the meaning that it conveys. And what, then, is this further meaning? A piece of information, one might be inclined to answer. However, to receive 'meanings' in the form of pieces of information is, of course, very far from reaching a sense of meaning in life. Inevitably, the path from finding out about the meaning of a word or a piece of information to 'constructing' an overriding meaning in events and in life is a long one.

This essay is going to deal with meaning in relation to (mainly) early symptoms of illness or disease. Symptoms are sensations, perceptions, from our body – and in psychiatric contexts also strange experiences – that we interpret as uncomfortable, peculiar, weird, threatening or even unbearable. When we start thinking about symptoms, we find ourselves occupied with a number of associated questions. For example, what, really, *are* illness and disease? When is a bodily perception understood as a symptom of illness? How may symptoms be combined and interpreted in a way that gives them meaning? Does a symptom really need to have a meaning? Can there be meaning on several different 'levels'? When does a symptom lead someone to seek help?

Even an attempt to start answering such chains of questions would lead us too far for our purposes here. Therefore we shall pass quickly over some of the associated issues, trusting that these have been sufficiently dealt with in other parts of Volume One. The focus of our attention will be those often fragmentary and emotionally disquieting experiences that are associated with certain perceptions from the body. This means that for the most part we shall omit psychiatric symptoms from the discussion, as these are not *primarily* concerned with the body and its functions. Our narratives – here, the experiences of Rachel and Geoff – will exemplify some of the arguments proposed. A few remarks will also be made about other narratives of illness and disease.

My wish is to explore how fruitful the use of a word like 'meaning' is when we attempt to understand or 'make sense of' what happens to a person who suddenly or gradually notices bodily signals – let us call them *bodily perceptions* – that are experienced as strange, unexpected and most often also worrying.[1] We are thus dealing with the very early phase of illness, its *status nascendi*. It may, however, not be the earliest stage of disease at all, as this concept is used to signify a pathological deviance in the functioning of the body, which frequently may go unnoticed by the individual.[2] It may also be worth noting that symptoms are not always new. They may have been there before, as uninteresting 'background' perceptions – but suddenly, through for example some new information or experience, they become interpreted in a new way, as threatening and alien.

THE APPEARANCE OF MEANING IN OUR LIVES

Let us first, perhaps somewhat boldly, attempt to say something about the role of meaning in our everyday life. There is a use of the word 'meaning' that refers to our experience that life makes sense, or adds up – that it is coherent and fruitful. This certainly does not require that every aspect of life, everything that happens to us and all of our actions, are meaningful in the sense of being intelligible, worthwhile and valuable. If I consider my life to be meaningful, this may be because, despite challenges and difficult elements, it gives me exactly the sense of coherence and control that is the basis for its meaningfulness. This *meaning in life* ought to be distinguished from my experience of the *meaning of life*. A sense of the meaning of life can hardly be a prerequisite for the conviction that my own life has a meaning for me (although one may suspect that it could contribute).

We attempt to construct an overall meaning in our lives in order to make sense of the world and its events and phenomena. But doesn't this just push the question a bit further away? What is it then to 'make sense of' something? (Is it perhaps synonymous with 'construct meaning', making our linguistic exercise circular?) We try again – we construct meaning because we need to orient ourselves in relation to the ongoing flux of events by which our lives are characterised. But 'construct'? A construction implies intent, conscious planning and goal-oriented action. To the extent that we experience a sense of meaning in our lives, few of us would be prepared to say that we 'planned' it in the sense that we intentionally created it. Isn't it rather that meaning is a sort of by-product of living – at least when our lives go on as they used to, when we are not interrupted by threatening or disruptive experiences? Meaning is then a dimension that in an enigmatic way emanates from our daily lives – and that makes them full and rich and worth living. Meaning makes our life world 'go together'.

In the following, I shall propose a way of looking at the notion of meaning as it relates to the situation when a person becomes ill. This means that we are asking for ways to understand and handle early symptoms of illness. I will suggest that when someone falls ill, meaning is closely connected to the experience of coherence, intelligibility, pattern recognition, and overall moral balance in the new situation. I thus take the dimensions of meaning, when confronted with early symptoms, to be threefold:

1 meaning on a basic causal level, where meaning appears when events can be causally linked (e.g. 'The pain is caused by obstructions in one or several vessels in the heart, leading to shortage of oxygen')

2 meaning as the appearance of an intelligible pattern on a more general level, in which case meaning presents itself when events and phenomena belong together in a way that creates a graspable pattern – partly causal and partly non-causal (e.g. 'My work has for a long time demanded more of me than I have been able to stand, which in combination with lack of physical exercise, occasional smoking and some genetic predisposition may have triggered the onset of the disease – and I now see that all of this is a part of the habits and desires that characterize my life as well as our time')

3 meaning on an existential level, appearing when our moral intuitions and our general reflections on our actions and on things that happen to us in our lives sum up in a way that seems coherent, understandable, 'makes

sense' – and to some reasonable degree 'harmonises' with our moral intuitions (e.g. 'I now realise that, due to lack of respect for myself, an excessive wish to please other people and a more or less constant feeling of guilt, I have neglected my needs both bodily and spiritual – and that the disease is the signal to me to reconsider my life in the light of this new understanding').

It will immediately be seen that these three forms of meaning are closely related. They all link factors – events, processes, states of body and mind – together in temporal chains. The first level is concerned with physical causality. The latter two involve agency and responsibility. They are based on a combination of scientific knowledge about the workings of the body and experiences from the life world, such as habits, desires, guilt and hope. The self-understanding that is involved in one dimension of meaning does not necessarily 'spill over' into another. I may receive medical explanations on level 1, but still be unable to connect this into a broader framework on level 2, and may be even further away from the meaning that appears on level 3. Explanations based on science are concerned with intellectual comprehension, basically accessible by anyone with intact cognitive capacities. Meaning in what may be called a moral/existential dimension is usually a much tougher task, usually takes a longer time and brings into focus the ill person's entire 'being-in-the-world.' No wonder that this dimension of meaning is often either avoided by clinical professionals as being too sensitive and too complex, or experienced by the ill person him- or herself as too heavily laden with guilt and self-reproach.

Of course, the gradual appearance of meaning in a situation with new and so far inexplicable perceptions from the body is to a large extent related to the increasing knowledge that the ill person will gain when they come into contact with professional care. In a society where medical services are easily accessible, the discomfort of not knowing usually leads the ill person to seek professional help. This will happen either when the symptoms are so oppressive and uncomfortable that they are hard to bear, or when, although more discrete and not in themselves unbearable, in the mind of the ill person the symptoms point in a dangerous direction, evoking fear of serious disease.

We need hardly be reminded that individuals react to this situation in strikingly different ways. People have widely varying resilience in this respect. A psychologist would perhaps relate this to differences in 'basic trust', the notion that Erik Eriksson uses to capture our degree of solid trust among all strains in life.[3] For some individuals, minor changes in bodily perception may be interpreted as potentially threatening and carrying grave meanings. In others, such shifts in the everyday perception of the body are just wiped away.[4] Some rush for help, while others reluctantly come when the situation is completely untenable. May we perhaps understand this in relation to our degree of attention to our bodily signals? Our central nervous system receives bodily signals all the time. It turns them into perceptions and interprets them – although the great majority of the afferent impulses are filtered away as unimportant, and therefore do not reach our consciousness. Just *how* our minds register and interpret the body is a fascinating and intriguing question indeed. To understand this we need to take both strictly physiological and also psychological and existential aspects into consideration.

THE NATURE OF SYMPTOMS

Let us return to the person who has just begun to experience peculiar and inexplicable sensations somewhere in their body. (It doesn't, of course, have to be 'somewhere', since many of the early symptoms we deal with in Volume One are 'non-localised' – where is dizziness, fatigue or nausea located?) We have already asked ourselves when these sensations become symptoms. Is it perhaps when they are either protracted or come back regularly, and at the same time are of a negative character? Should we say that a sensation from the body that is not in some sense negative and that therefore does not entail discomfort is perhaps not a symptom?

In Lars Gustafsson's *The Death of a Beekeeper*, the narrator, who is a retired teacher living with his dog in the countryside, starts to experience abdominal pain, which gradually increases over the weeks from being rather diffuse to becoming intense, throbbing and terrifying. The beekeeper walks around the landscape with his dog, and at those times when the pain is intense it textures his whole experience of the landscape around him. Gustafsson's beekeeper is inevitably preoccupied by questions of meaning – they permeate his very existence. He writes in his diary (*my translation*):[5]

> Why exactly me?
> Why exactly me mortal?
> Why exactly me this pain?
> Why exactly me identical with this pain?
> Why exactly me identical with someone who feels this pain?
> Why . . .

Which emotions do we associate with most early symptoms? Normally, as just noted, we can hardly call a pleasant sensation a symptom.[6] Discomfort most often accompanies symptoms, and may perhaps under some circumstances constitute a symptom in itself. We experience surprise, certainly, and almost always worry, sometimes verging on fear. It seems to be typical of early symptoms that they are unpleasant both 'in themselves' and also for what they do to us (e.g. by preventing us from doing the things that we like to do). These two aspects of discomfort are often inextricably linked. It is worth bearing in mind that many of the symptoms that send people to doctors are perhaps not as uncomfortable in themselves as they are for what they are thought to mean for the future, as they are interpreted as potential threats to future health, and hence in a sense are loaded with future discomfort.[7]

Are we entitled to say that the negative emotional taint on symptoms goes away when meaning is established – even if the sensation is still there? To put it another way, is establishing the meaning of a symptom the same as freeing it of its negative emotional content? Yes, it seems as if it is, at least sometimes. If a bodily sensation is uncomfortable because of its threatening character (and hence is a 'symptom'), and if I am assured that it is insignificant, not related to future disease, the perception ceases to be a 'symptom.' The meaning – the relief – that the reassurance gives me changes the character of the perception.

However, if I am in chronic pain from a joint disorder and if I am able to make some kind of meaning out of my situation, can my pain then be turned into something that is not (entirely) negative? Many of us have met people who experience chronic pain and who declare that their lives are full of meaning despite the pain. But this can hardly mean that *the pain itself* is meaningful, but rather that their lives are meaningful *despite* the pain. Is it perhaps even self-contradictory to talk about a meaningful pain?[8]

Let us consider Rachel in our narrative. She is 10 years old. Her knowledge of diseases is of course extremely limited. Thirst is a perception, a sensation, that she cannot be expected to associate with any specific disorder. Had she been 20, it is far more likely that she herself would, at an early stage of her symptoms, have been able to make a preliminary meaning out of her tormenting experience through the concept of diabetes (what I here call 'level (1) meaning').

Rachel is thirsty, unbearably so. The thirst is like an alien force invading her life – disruptive, cruel and merciless. She gives in to it, but this only makes things worse. By mostly drinking sweet drinks she slips into a vicious circle of increased hyperglycaemia, which can only end in a coma. The days leading up to her collapse seem like a nightmare. The thirst – or rather the situation of being desperately thirsty – is literally meaningless to Rachel. It has no function, it has no origin, and it plays no constructive role in her life. The only 'meaning' of this symptom is incessantly to demand its own satisfaction, only to come back after a short while, in a never-ending devilish race. A bodily symptom as seriously disruptive as this turns life upside down. Rachel cannot go on living her life as she has been used to. The symptom is 'imperialistic', as it forces almost all other aspects of her life to succumb to its rule. Whatever Rachel does, the thirst is there. She cannot escape.

Can meaning be given to such an insatiable bodily sensation? Ordinarily the point of perceiving thirst is that the thirsty person drinks, and the meaning is given by the fact that there was a lack of fluid in the body which is now corrected. Meaning is in that case associated with action, and the proof that the meaning was correctly interpreted is that the perception of thirst goes away, in this case after drinking – and that the body is brought back to a situation of balance. But what if the thirst just goes on and on, as it does for Rachel? The insatiably thirsty person suffers, partly because the sensation is unpleasant in itself, and partly because of the total inexplicability of it all. None of the dimensions discussed above that could have provided a meaning in her situation are there. There is no causal explanation, no context in which to fit the thirst. It won't go away, however much she drinks. It makes her body feel threatening and alien. There is no name for it that can render trust and consolation, and there is less and less hope for a future without its dictatorial reign.

In a later volume we shall see what happens when Rachel is treated for her coma and when she is informed about the disease, how it works, and what consequences it will have for her life. She will then certainly have taken *one* of the important steps towards establishing a meaning in her new life situation. She will in some ways be relieved by the diagnosis, despite the serious nature of her disorder. We may well imagine Rachel's emotional turmoil when the word 'diabetes' is first uttered to her, when she is in hospital recovering from her diabetic coma. Relief will be mixed with sorrow and fear. Still, to know is better than not to know. The previously unknown danger now at least takes a shape and is given a name. It can be handled. But meaningfulness will still be far off.

Meaning in early illness is, as we can see from the above discussion, closely connected with the small word 'Why?' It is the individual's struggle with this 'Why?' that largely determines how the search for meaning will proceed. The answers will be sought inside the ill person, by comparing the symptoms with personal experiences and knowledge. Sooner or later, however, when the person has come to think of the perceptions as communicable symptoms – and to see that something may be gained by communicating them – people around will be brought in and hence become parts of the struggle for meaning. A friend may be trusted and may tell of similar sensations that turned out to be completely innocent – or a relative may give the advice to seek help as soon as possible, because this whole resembles something that she knows as harmful and dangerous.

We may think of the role of narrative here. Nowadays, much is made of the fact that narratives play such a vital role in our lives. We are reminded that the dimension of meaning in life is frequently structured by narrative. But what does this mean in the case of symptoms? Symptoms have a start, they go on and lead to further events and actions, they temper our daily lives, they develop in time and change character, they go away and they come back. Narratives unfold over time, as do symptoms. Narratives have an end, as do symptoms usually. Narratives are able to capture our existence as, at the same time, bodily and spiritual beings. Symptoms comprise these two aspects. Integrating symptoms into a story (which may be more or less extensive) is probably a way of giving them meaning. But how may this be done?

If I ask myself 'Why do I have this accursed throbbing pain in my back?', my wish for a medical explanation is of course also triggered by a hope for a remedy – or at least for confirmation that this is not a tumour or something else that is *really* dangerous. If we know *why* (in the scientific sense of the word), we will often know *how* (to treat). The general truth of this is not changed by the fact that it is not always the case. If I am given solid enough reason to believe that my symptoms will go away as a result of treatment, and if this treatment does not seem to be too threatening, then the urge to establish a meaningful coexistence with the symptoms may seem less pressing. I can go on looking at it as a dreadful episode from which luckily I was saved by a successful treatment. Diagnosis is, in these cases, followed by relief, because it offers full cure. But the delay until diagnosis will still often be full of unanswered questions.

The wish for a medical, meaning-giving explanation is certainly often ambivalent. I may hope that a diagnosis of a tumour can be excluded, but at the same time I fear that it will be confirmed, and I fear this so strongly that I resent the visit to the doctor. Jen, the exhausted wife of a stroke-ridden husband in our narrative, of course wants to know why there is blood in her sputum when she coughs – and yet she seems to want to remain ignorant. How common this dilemma is, this Janus face of knowledge in our lives!

If the early symptoms are indicators of a chronic disabling disorder, the situation will be very different. The first challenge may be the same. But here there is no immediate consolation in diagnosis, apart from the not unimportant relief of simply knowing. The evil will not go away. It will remain, as in Rachel's case, where the most dangerous phase of her diabetes will be checked by insulin injections and the disease kept under reasonable control, but her life will be more or less transformed by its presence.

We have noted the crucial role of '*Why* questions' when symptoms appear.

But this 'Why?' means more than just a wish to know about a bodily dysfunction. As indicated by our tentative dimensions of meaning, to know why is also a longing for a more general intelligibility, and for moral consolation. Rachel, we can be sure, will many times ask herself – and occasionally also others – why it was that *she* got this dreadful disorder and not her friends or her brother? She will certainly not be fully satisfied by answers based on epidemiology – for example, that the reason she fell ill is to be seen in a number of contributing 'risk factors', of which she happened to have some in a sufficient combination to make her vulnerable and finally ill. She will go on asking about the justice of this, about contingency and chance and fate. The extent to which Rachel will suffer will be dependent on her answers to these questions – and these answers will largely depend on her interactions with important individuals around her. We may perhaps also say that it is her opportunity to integrate her symptoms successfully into her life story that determines the outcome of her coexistence with the disease.

Leo Tolstoy's short story *The Death of Ivan Ilyich* exemplifies the urgent need for moral reconciliation when facing very serious disease and death.[9] Ivan is a successful civil servant in tsarist Russia. He marries, has two children, establishes a career, and gradually loses contact with his wife and family. One day he starts to experience an abdominal pain, which is mild at first, but gradually gets worse. After a short delay the doctors are asked for advice. They realise what this is about – an abdominal tumour – but Ivan is not told. As a result, the symptoms go on living their own cruel life, while Ivan is held in ignorance of their significance. He is efficiently obstructed from developing any meaning about what is going on, and from integrating the sensations in his stomach into his personal story. No 'Why?' question is answered. At the climax of the story, Ivan's pain is so intractable that he can no longer avoid the realisation that he is going to succumb to this 'whatever-it-is.' He starts screaming, a horrifying scream of fear, grief and anger – and his screaming goes on for days. Is Ivan's screaming a desperate expression of the realisation that his life has already been lost, devoid of any meaning, long before the disease is going to end it? If so, who could restore some sense of overall meaning to Ivan before he goes into that dark night? A servant boy is the one who will do this, in a deeply moving scene – and Ivan's life ends in a brittle consolation with himself, his disorder and his life, as it became.

Ivan Ilyich's story perhaps tells us that when serious symptoms strike a person who is already in grave difficulties in finding meaning in his life, the symptoms may be even more meaningless and threatening. They may be the reminders of this lack of meaning. They may be the cruel spotlights upon the realisation that life has been without meaning, useless, and of no value.

In psychiatric language this is the state of depression, and in existential terms it is the state of despair.

On the other hand, symptoms may prompt a search for an absent meaning in one's life. A breakthrough to new possibilities may emerge.

SYMPTOM AND SIGN

Let us return to the person with early symptoms, and for a while adopt a phenomenological perspective on health and illness. Key notions in the phenomenology of the body are the *life world* and the *lived body*. The former refers to our everyday conceptions of the world around us, as they are formed when our consciousness intentionally directs itself towards shifting phenomena. The lived body may be seen as a crucial constituent of this life world, and possibly the most crucial. The lived body is the point of departure of all our knowledge of the world. It is *as* bodies, and *with* and *through* our bodies, that we interact with the world.[10] In the words of philosopher Kay Toombs, 'The body is not an object akin to other physical, animate objects in the world, but, rather, the medium through which, and by means of which, I apprehend the world and interact with it.'[11]

Early symptoms of illness create a rupture in this 'taken-for-granted' relationship to the world. The body, which is under ordinary circumstances so self-evidently identical with our self, changes character, and becomes estranged, alien and not to be trusted. We are not at home in our bodies any more, which means that neither are we at home in ourselves. The phenomenologist Fredrik Svenaeus, inspired by the philosopher Gadamer, views this as the very essence of illness – an experience of homelessness that is the result of a basic change in our perceptions of our bodies.[12] This change creates obstacles to our plans and aspirations, and suffering is the result of this, together with the direct physical consequences (e.g. pain, nausea, itching, fatigue, etc.) that constitute the symptoms.

In his collection of essays entitled *The Enigma of Health*, the above-mentioned Hans-Georg Gadamer writes about the loss of health (something that we would usually equate with being ill) as an *absence*.[13] He also interestingly notes that pain and suffering have a tendency to turn our attention inwards. This may be experienced as an alienation from the world, as when Rainer Maria Rilke, in a late poem, seriously ill with a blood malignancy, writes about his wish to be 'out there.' This certainly does not only mean physically, but also captures a sense of no longer belonging to the community of living beings, and of being expelled from the world.

Phenomenology may help us to understand some of the early reactions to symptoms. It also helps us to see the interesting difference between what is in medical literature usually called a sign and a symptom. Let us think about a woman who one morning notices a lump in her left breast. She is convinced that this lump was not there before. At once, of course, her head is filled with chaotic questions. Is this a cancer? If it is, will I die from it? Could it be something else that isn't dangerous? How do I handle this? Will I have to wait long to know? Whom do I tell?

Is the lump a symptom? In a sense yes, it is, as it is subjectively experienced and gives rise to a number of questions. However, in stark contrast to the pain or vertigo or nausea, the lump is also inter-subjectively detectable. No one will see my nausea (although certainly people will often see some of the associated somatic reactions, such as pallor and sweating). It is, in this sense, strictly mine. I can't ask for immediate confirmation from anyone else. The lump is different. It is there. The lump *is* the disorder as it presents itself through a sign. In the case of nausea, it is rather as if this symptom is *pointing to* the disorder. The symptom is a clue to the existence of disease, but not the disease itself. (Although admittedly signs like pallor, tremor, jaundice, etc. are also pointing to diseases rather than being diseases in themselves.)

In the case of the woman with a lump, the knowledge of a bodily change that has not yet caused any harm 'triggers' a chain of questions and causes deep fear. It will also entail a shift in her perception of her body. It is now both her most obvious reality – her basic source of identity – and at the same time something alien and threatening, something that is not herself any more. In her body there is a growth that is not *she*, that is something else, an intruder. She may even start to develop peculiar sensations from the area with the lump, indicating how powerful the interpretive activity of the mind is for our perceptions of our bodies.

We see that the detection (in this case tactile) by the woman herself of a bodily change results in basically the same loss of evident meaning and trust as does the experience of a symptom like nausea or fatigue. However, as we have already noted, these latter sensations are non-directed, global, diffuse and non-measurable. This may make them more difficult to cope with, in the sense that they are less easily communicable. The woman with a breast lump *knows* that anyone else would feel what she does if they investigated her breast. The man with severe and protracted fatigue knows that the symptom is exclusively *his*, and thus in an important sense incommunicable. Jen, in our narrative, has streaks of blood in her sputum – a grave sign in medicine. She knows that this may be dangerous. She is ambivalent about what she knows will follow from her contacts with her doctor. Her problem is *recognised* but has still not been handled.

We may put this another way. Signs have a higher degree of inter-subjectivity than do symptoms. Signs are often measurable, and are possible to depict and present in a material sense. This may lead to the unfortunate and misguided conclusion that symptoms without signs are less real. Of course they are not. However, giving meaning to symptoms may, for exactly this reason, be more difficult. A symptom without any accompanying sign – either directly or on laboratory investigation – will face a greater risk of not being confirmed by those significant others from whom confirmation is so crucial.[14] It will certainly make contacts with medical professionals more complicated and risky. One may wonder whether this does not sometimes lead to aggravation of the invisible symptoms, in an unconscious and almost desperate attempt to 'convince' the world of their existence.[15]

SYMPTOMS AS CREATORS OF MEANING

This chapter has the title 'Giving meaning to symptoms.' This is based on an almost intuitive assumption, presumably shared by most of us, that symptoms come first – I become dizzy for several hours and almost immediately attempt to make sense of this uncomfortable experience – and that a sense of meaningfulness is something which will hopefully emerge from this challenge. We 'cope with' symptoms, but would rather do without them. But what if this is not always the case? What if a loss of meaning, or serious threat to meaning, *precedes* symptoms, and thus in a way sometimes *causes* them? If the way that we communicate symptoms arouses the attention of those significant others who surround us, if this communicated content ('I do not feel well – please notice me, help me and take care of me') in a peculiar way actually restores a lost sense of meaning in my life, could it not then be that I am sometimes tempted to 'fabricate' these symptoms? Certainly I do not do this as a conscious agent, but rather as a gradual, invisible, disguised process of coming to terms with a situation that threatens to become, or already is, unbearable.

Something like this has been proposed by a number of observers, one of them being the Swedish physician Olle Hellström.[16] It follows from his way of thinking that if a sense of meaning (coherence, intelligibility, moral trust) can be regained in life *without* the symptoms – which anyway in the longer term threaten to destroy any meaningful existence – they will go away. But of course, if this is the case, it would be preferable for this insight to emanate from the ill person him- or herself, rather than being a more or less intrusive suspicion on the part of the doctor.

It is clear that symptoms, under certain circumstances, may be a risky source of a new, powerful and even tempting life-meaning. Recall Hans Castorp, who accompanied his cousin to the sanatorium in Davos, in Thomas Mann's great novel *The Magic Mountain*.[17] Hans has some very mild and inconspicuous symptoms like a low-grade fever, a slightly elevated pulse, and red bloom on the cheeks. Step by step, almost invisibly, his identity changes under the influence of the sanatorium's atmosphere and the charismatic power of Dr Behrens, its chief physician. Hans' way of looking upon himself – in a sense, his life meaning – is reconstructed from being a healthy young student to being a person with a serious and at the time usually incurable disease, tuberculosis. All the symbolic associations of tuberculosis and the sanatorium – with eroticism, with creativity, with sensuality, with a slower pace of time, and with a world secluded from the turmoil of the outer realities – half-consciously and subconsciously drag Hans into this world of disease, and permeate him with a strong and seductive sense of meaning.

RECOGNITION

Finally, I would like to return to the crucial moment when a person with symptoms turns to someone for help. Isn't this the almost archetypical situation in which we fully realise how deeply related we are to others and how embedded our lives are in a social context? And when we also realise that ability to discover meaning in threatening events crucially depends on the outcome of the encounter with others? 'I just cannot handle this any more, help me' – this common phrase entails both a trust that there *is* help to get and that there are people *willing* to give us this help. John Berger has, in his wonderful book about country doctor John Sassall, pointed to one factor that perhaps more than anything else determines the outcome of this encounter.[18] It is *recognition*. Recognition here has the double meaning of showing to the ill person that I really *know* that she experiences what she does experience, and also that this is something that I recognise – *I have seen it before, and because of this professional experience, I know what to do*. The ill person's trust that this will happen when she seeks help is the one factor that, more than any other, enables her to reach some kind of meaning in early illness:

> Most unhappiness is like illness in that it too exacerbates a sense of uniqueness. All frustration magnifies its own dissimilarity and so nourishes itself. . . . It is a question of failing to find any confirmation in the outside world. The lack of confirmation leads to a sense of futility. And this sense of futility is the essence of loneliness: for, despite the horrors of history, the existence of other men

always promises the possibility of purpose. Any example offers hope. But the conviction of being unique destroys all examples.[19]

REFERENCES

1 I use the word 'perception' here as basically synonymous with 'sensation.' Both perception and sensation, in my terminology, lie a step before we consciously start to interpret. To put it another way, a bodily perception becomes a symptom through a certain kind of interpretation. However, it is hard to think of any perception from the body that causes distress that is not *almost* immediately the object of the mind's searching to understand its origin, role and significance.

2 A tempting and very common example would be increased blood pressure at levels which are thought to be dangerous, in the short or long term, for the individual. Most often, this hypertension is not accompanied by any symptoms whatsoever. That is, the individual's perceptions of their body are not changed due to this physiological abnormality.

3 Eriksson EH. *The Life Cycle Completed: a review*. New York: Norton; 1982.

4 A common although drastic example of this is hypochondria. The hypochondriac 'fabricates' symptoms by an incessant introspection accompanied by an inclination to think the worst of any minor signal.

5 Gustafsson L. *En Biodlares Död*. Stockholm: Norstedts; 1984. p. 113.

6 Or may we perhaps occasionally? Dostoyevsky writes about the pleasure in the aura preceding the epileptic seizure, and may we not sometimes experience certain sensations from the skin – like tickling – as almost enjoyable (at least for a while)?

7 It may be that the more medical care is occupied with risk management, with detecting risks for diseases at an early stage, the more people will tend to look upon bodily sensations as potentially threatening and consequently as 'symptoms.'

8 In his book *The Culture of Pain*, Morris insists that modern scientific medicine has made it almost impossible to look upon pain as meaningful, thereby putting a heavy burden on those whose pain will not go away with the help of conventional medical measures.

9 Tolstoy L. *The Death of Ivan Ilych*. Letchworth: Bradda Books; 1966.

10 Bullington J. *The Mysterious Life of the Body: a new look at psychosomatics*. Linköping: Linköping Studies in Arts and Science; 1999; Rudebeck C-E. General practice and the dialogue of clinical practice: on symptoms, symptom presentations and bodily empathy. *Scand J Prim Health Care*. 1992; **Suppl. 1**.

11 Toombs K. Introduction: phenomenology and medicine. In: Toombs K, editor. *Handbook of Phenomenology and Medicine*. Dordrecht: Kluwer Academic Publishers; 2001. p. 5.

12 Svenaeus F. *The Hermeneutics of Medicine and the Phenomenology of Health: steps towards a philosophy of medical practice*. Linköping: Linköping Studies in Arts and Science; 1999.

13 Gadamer H-G. *The Enigma of Health: the art of healing in a scientific age*. Cambridge: Polity Press; 1996.

14 A woman with chronic fatigue syndrome once replied, when I had somewhat naively

complimented her on her rested appearance, that '. . . it is exactly this that is the heart of the problem.'

15 If this is so, it is easy to understand the crucial importance of a confirming attitude on the part of health professionals when patients present with diffuse symptoms – 'illness without disease.'

16 Hellström O. Health promotion and the clinical dialogue. *Patient Educ Counsel.* 1995; **25**: 247–56.

17 Mann T. *Der Zauberberg.* Frankfurt: S Fischer Verlag; 2002 (originally published in 1934).

18 Berger J. *A Fortunate Man: the story of a country doctor.* New York: Vintage Books; 1997 (originally published in 1967).

19 Ibid., pp. 74–5.

Index